INVESTING IN YOUR HEALTH

A Pharmacist's Guide to Choosing Natural Products

GK SISKA RPH, PHARMD

To Erika,

I'm wishing you great success in all areas of life..... especially great Health.

With Love,

Gunda

CONTENTS

1. Introduction: Health is Wealth   1
2. Vitamins and Minerals   11
3. Correcting Excessive Oxidative Damage   33
4. Optimizing the Gut   45
5. Reducing Inflammation with Natural Products   57
6. Strengthening the Immune System   67
7. The Mind/Body Connection   83
8. Detoxing the Body of Chemical Disruptors   99
9. Optimizing Blood Sugars, Appetite Control, and Weight Loss   113
10. Energy Precursors Are an Emerging Area of Medicine   131
11. Hormones and Longevity   139
12. Understanding how these Ten Areas Affect Our Health   153

References   161

This book is dedicated to all the people who search for better health, energy and vitality. I humbly offer up the information and insights that I have accumulated over the decades during my work as a pharmacist. I believe the more we understand, the more we are able to understand in the future. There is so much information out there and more information is still coming in. My hope is to get people started learning about their health and on the path to a better, healthier life.

Special thanks to Wilfrid Koponen for all his help with this book. You are a great friend, author, and mentor. Also, thanks to Caitlin Mollison, Kristen Crossley, and Colleen Hall who had a huge impact on my development as a medical writer. Thank you for the years of leading me by example.

①

INTRODUCTION: HEALTH IS WEALTH

Cracking the Code: The Future of Longevity Medicine

Discovering longevity genes and activating them gave us hope that we could extend our lives. The Foxxo genes and the Sirt2 genes are thought to be responsible for great health and a long life—the kind of health that would allow people to drink and smoke to their delight yet reap no adverse consequences. People without these genes, on the other hand, suffer premature negative health consequences despite eating healthy foods and exercising appropriately. Activating these genes is like activating an internal maintenance team that fixes almost any damage in our body before bad health sets in. When scientists discovered resveratrol and rapamycin, we had glimpses of turning these and other genes on in animals and other primitive life forms. But translating this information to humans has been more difficult.

Finding optimal health and slowing the aging process down is like cracking the code that opens up a combination safe full of energy, feeling good, looking good, pleasant mood, restful sleep, and improved libido. The combination is different for every person because our health is so individualized. We must be our own superintendents. Our minds must be the supervisor of the maintenance teams. The maintenance workers must be the appropriate whole foods, amino acids, medicinal oils, vitamins, minerals, nutraceuticals, and drugs. We must use our minds to control our health and to mimic these longevity genes. We must use all the tools in our toolbox if we want to extend our lives and enjoy optimal quality of life for as long as possible. We must use medicinal diets first, natural products second, drugs and hormones third. All these approaches should be based on medical studies and in alignment with what up-to-date medical experts say.

There are ten areas in which we can intervene with natural products to bring us back into alignment with the vibrant health of our youth. The natural products used to optimize these ten areas of health are the combination codes to opening up a vault fault full of energy, health, great mood, and looking and feel

ONE: VITAMINS AND MINERALS

good. This combination code is based on our genetics and our lifestyle. It is different for everyone.

ONE: VITAMINS AND MINERALS

There are overt and subclinical vitamin deficiencies. Most people over 50 have some sort of vitamin deficiency due to malabsorption of nutrients and lifestyle. We know these deficiencies are real because they show up in blood tests as low levels. The most common deficiencies are vitamin D, magnesium, and phosphate. Sometimes they show up as disease symptoms. The B vitamin deficiencies are commonly causes of neurological problems, such as Wernicke's encephalitis, migraines, and other neuropathies.

To maintain excellent health, our vitamin levels must be in the perfect range—not too high and not too low. Who is at risk of falling out of the perfect zone? I write about signs and symptoms that can manifest when these individual and specific levels fall out of range.

What are overt symptoms and subclinical symptoms of vitamin deficiencies? Subclinical vitamin deficiencies mimic signs of old age, but they are not signs of old age. They include frequent colds and infections, low energy levels, brain fog, and other mysterious symptoms. Overt symptoms of deficiencies are obvious signs that medical practitioners can detect, such as rickets, scurvy, neurologic damage, pellagra, and anemia, to name a few.

We must dispel the myth that more vitamins are necessarily better. When a low vitamin level is restored to normal, miraculous things happen. When a normal vitamin level is elevated, good things rarely happen, and sometimes, bad things happen

TWO: CORRECTING EXCESSIVE OXIDATIVE STATES WITH ANTIOXIDANTS BEFORE DAMAGE SETS IN

What is an antioxidant? Imagine hydrogen peroxide poured onto an open wound. The liquid forms bubbles as it consumes dead or infected flesh. The right amount cleans up the wound. But if the hydrogen peroxide solution is too strong and excessive, damage to healthy tissue also takes place. Our bodies normally make the perfect amount of natural hydrogen peroxide to keep our tissues clean. However, too much or too little of this natural hydrogen peroxide is not good for us. Studies have shown that in healthy individuals, antioxidant use can have negative effects, but in certain disease states, especially diabetes, antioxidants can improve health.

THREE: THE GUT, THE BEGINNING OF GOOD HEALTH

Many doctors believe that a healthy gut is the foundation of good health. There are six ways our gut affects our health. Biochemical reactions take place in the gut, the immune system is located here, leaky gut contributes to systemic inflammation, latent infections or dysbiosis can occur here, toxin and waste removal occur in the gut, and the gut extracts nutrients from the foods that we are digesting. Which natural products optimize the gut and keep it running in top condition?

FOUR: CONTROLLING SYSTEMIC INFLAMMATION WITH NATURAL SUPPLEMENTS

Many antiaging experts believe systemic inflammation accelerates bad health into a downward spiral. Systemic inflammation is also thought to be responsible for body aches, swelling, puffiness under the eyes, skin eruptions, and redness—to name just a few things.

But what about heart disease, cancer and diabetes? The American Heart Association, American Diabetes Association, and The National Cancer Institute/National Institutes of Health are all looking at this link for possible future interventions.

Natural products have been shown to reduce low-grade inflammation. I will discuss this in detail.

FIVE: FORTIFYING THE IMMUNE SYSTEM BY USING NATURAL PRODUCTS WITH ANTIVIRAL PROPERTIES

For a long and healthy life, it is essential to have an immune system that is in perfect balance. An immune system out of balance is associated with autoimmune diseases and frequent infections. We must support and develop the immune system but not throw it off balance with the wrong types of products. We are fighting an invisible war against pathogens. We must first have a strong immune system and then use antiviral products to speed recovery and prevent viral infections during epidemics. Bacterial, fungal, parasitic, and serious viral infections require drugs. But the common cold and flu viruses can be treated with specific natural products that are readily available on the market. People need to keep up with changing information about products coming on and off the market as new findings alter previous best practices.

SIX: THE MIND/BODY CONNECTION

The mind/body connection is real, and it goes both ways. A brain on fire with inflammation and other diseases will sabotage our thoughts and cause a downward spiral of physical health. Which products keep the mind balanced with abundant neurochemicals and proper blood flow to the brain?

SEVEN: DETOXING

Toxins sabotage our health, so keeping the liver and kidney healthy so that they can help us to detoxify is essential. Our bodies have four methods by which to remove toxins: the liver; the kidneys; the intestines; and skin, hair, and nails. Toxins are called enzyme disruptors and hormonal disruptors. They disrupt the biochemistry in our bodies and sabotage optimal health and energy production. What does heavy metal poisoning look like so that people can recognize if it occurs?

EIGHT: APPETITE CONTROL, MEDICINAL DIETS, AND CONTROLLING BLOOD SUGAR

The best predictor of health and longevity is a test called Hemoglobin A1c. The number from this test is closely related to elevated blood sugar levels that damage our cells and tissues microscopically. Amino acids, medicinal oils, fiber products, and probiotics can help us take control of our appetite. Which products can affect insulin resistance, as well as controlling and lowering blood-sugar levels?

NINE: ENERGY AND NATURAL SUPPLEMENTS THAT BUILD ADENOSINE TRI-PHOSPHATE (ATP)

Energy is the essence of life. As we age, scientists can measure a reduction in the quantity of certain energy-related chemicals in our bodies. Some doctors believe that restoring these energy-related chemicals to normal levels would allow the body to make repairs, avoid disease, avoid bad health, and strengthen the immune system.

The epic article "Hallmarks of Aging" (López-Otín et al., 2013) discussed mitochondrial dysfunction. In addition to that, we can learn from treating people with diseases that involve energy production, such as congenital mitochondrial dysfunction, heart failure, and certain brain-related anomalies.

TEN: HORMONALLY ACTIVE NATURAL PRODUCTS AND LONGEVITY MEDICINE

Hormones are like vitamins. They must be in the healthy zone. Levels that are too high or too low cause problems. Some hormones cause cell growth, while others cause cells to break down. With the passage of time, we want continued cell growth to maintain bone mass, muscle mass, brain mass, strong tendons, and strong internal organs. Too much cell breakdown is bad. Too much cell growth is also bad. We need the right balance of cell growth to maintain a youthful homeostasis. Which natural products alter our hormone levels? Which are the most important hormones that affect our longevity: the parathyroid hormone and Vitamin D, insulin, the growth and repair hormone, testosterone, estrogen, progesterone, DHEA, and others.

CONCLUSION

It is my belief that there is no single product that will yield overall good health for everyone. Natural products yield good health by correcting a problem or an imbalance. How and when we can use natural products is a complex picture that is slowly coming into focus for us. We will continue to gather more knowledge and information. I look forward to sharing my knowledge with the world and listening to others' thoughts on the subject.

2

VITAMINS AND MINERALS

Some experts say that vitamins are a waste of money and THAT healthy people don't need to take dietary supplements to stay healthy. Other experts say that you can prevent certain cancers and cardiovascular diseases through taking specific supplements, regardless of your current health status. These experts espouse views that are polar opposites, and probably nothing will make these two groups agree. Even if they read the same empirical study, they will come to different conclusions, no matter what the data show. If the facts are undeniably against their cause, they will claim that the study was poorly designed or had inconclusive evidence. So where does that leave us—the people in search of the truth who wish to optimize personal health? **There is a pattern.**

When a vitamin that is deficient is restored to normal levels, miraculous things happen:

- Life expectancy goes up.
- Chronic wounds heal.
- Energy levels increase.
- Vision is preserved.
- Skin and hair glow.
- The immune system gets stronger.
- Infections are more easily resisted.

However, if you take a normal vitamin level and elevate it with synthetic supplements, good things do not happen. Sometimes, bad things happen, especially for people who are frail or weak.

Consider studies of multivitamin use. Undernourished, impoverished men in China who took a multivitamin lived longer (Blot et al., 1993). Well-nourished doctors in America who took a multivitamin did not live longer than did well-nourished doctors who did not take a multivitamin supplement, possibly because they were already in a peak state of health (Muntwyler et al., 2002).

Children in third-world countries whose lives were being cut short due to infectious diseases, such as pneumonia and infectious diarrhea, lived longer when given zinc supplements (Black, 2003). U.S. pharmaceutical companies have capitalized on this correlation by marketing zinc products to consumers to prevent or reduce the duration of the common cold. But does taking zinc supplements have the same effect in the U.S. for well-nourished Americans? No, not so much. Our life expectancy does not go up as it does in studies of third-world children. The pattern repeats for energy levels and iron deficiencies. When given iron pills, people who are anemic from an iron deficiency get more energy, and their anemia goes away.

We need to keep vitamin levels within an optimal natural range. It's similar to blood sugar, food, water, oxygen, sunshine, and sleep: either too much or too little can be dangerous. It is a pattern that is repeated over and over in nature and revealed in the medical literature. If you picked any vitamin study in the literature and read it carefully, you would notice that the vitamin only worked if the person had a deficiency to begin with. Sometimes, that is not disclosed, and then the results are muddy. But with careful analysis of the data, you can learn that the vitamin never or rarely worked when the person in the study was properly nourished.

Fortunately, laboratories are now developing the equipment to measure vitamin levels in our blood to see whether they are in the healthy range. Just as doctors currently measure sodium, potassium, and magnesium, one day we should be able to monitor levels for all vitamins.

THE SECRET TO GETTING GOOD RESULTS FROM VITAMINS IS KNOWING WHEN TO USE THEM

Vitamins should be used when people show overt symptoms, subclinical symptoms, or demonstrate known risk factors for vitamin deficiencies. (See Table 1. Who Benefits from Taking Vitamins?)

INVESTING IN YOUR HEALTH

Table 1. Who Benefits from Taking Vitamins?	
People Who:	**Can Benefit from Taking:**
Eat poor or impoverished diets typical of third-world countries or are in prisons or similar institutions	multivitamin, B12, vitamin D, and vitamin C (depending on how severe the diet and condition)
Do not eat fruits or vegetables	multivitamin, magnesium
Are strict vegetarians	vitamin B12, Zinc
Have had gastric bypass surgery	multivitamin with iron, vitamin C, vitamin B12, vitamin D, magnesium
Suffer from Crohn's disease, colitis, or celiac disease	multivitamin, iron, calcium, vitamin B12, vitamin D, magnesium
Regularly consume alcohol	multivitamin, vitamin B12, folic acid, thiamin, magnesium
Are on lifelong medications for chronic conditions, such as heartburn, diabetes, or seizures	vitamin B12, vitamin D, magnesium, multivitamin
Are pregnant	multivitamin, extra folic acid, maybe calcium, iron
Are >50 (Lundberg, 2015; McBride, 2000; Tangpricha et al., 2016)	vitamin B12 & D, magnesium.
Athletes who run marathons or are in constant motion for long periods of time who are unable to restore their vitamin levels through diet (Hemilä et al., 2013; Vitamin C, 2014)	vitamin C, multivitamin, vitamin B complex
Smoke or those who are exposed to second-hand smoke (Institute, 2000)	vitamin C
Are on dialysis	Depends on lab work — never take any new vitamin without consulting your doctor

SUMMARY OF RISK FACTORS FOR VITAMIN DEFICIENCIES

• People who have conditions involving the gastrointestinal tract, gastritis, GERD, swallowing issues, chronic nausea and vomiting, gastroparesis, gastric bypass, chronic diarrhea for any reason, colitis, and especially celiac disease

- People who eat a limited diet. Those living in third-world countries, people who are institutionalized (in prisons, group homes, nursing homes, etc.), picky eaters, vegans, vegetarians, long-term ketogenic dieters, people with anorexia or an eating disorder
- People with genetic defects involving their biochemistry pathways. We cannot always identify these defects and are still discovering more about them. But 60 percent of people with sickle-cell anemia also have a zinc deficiency. There are also phenotypes involving vitamin C, and D.
- People with frequent exposure to toxins and hazardous chemicals. The U.S. Task Force for the Institutes of Medicine (IOM) of the National Academies (formerly National Academy of Sciences) said that smokers have lower levels of vitamin C and should take a vitamin C supplement. People who drink alcohol frequently often have multiple deficiencies, particularly B vitamins. People can have drug-induced vitamin deficiencies from prescription drugs (NIH, ODS, 2020a).

VITAMIN D AND THE DISCOVERY OF SUB-CLINICAL DEFICIENCIES

Recently it was discovered that vitamin D is an insidious vitamin deficiency. That means that there are people walking around with this deficiency who don't know that they have it. They may think that their mysterious symptoms (such as brain fog, low energy, frequent infections, weakness, unsteady gait, and many other adverse effects) are a result of old age, but these mysterious symptoms can actually be a result of a low vitamin D level. Fortunately, doctors who think outside the box discovered that elevating vitamin D levels cured or alleviated many of these symptoms.

Prior to this discovery, vitamin D deficiencies were only associated with bad bones, as in rickets in children and osteomalacia in adults. Now we know that vitamin D does so much more than keep our bones healthy. Vitamin D is now being called a hormone because there are vitamin D receptors and activating enzymes on almost every cell in the body. As we age, our bodies become less efficient at making vitamin D.

Vitamin D starts out as a cholesterol molecule, which we can call vitamin D1. Near the skin's surface, it gets zapped by sunshine and becomes vitamin D2 (ergocalciferol). Then it gets transformed by activating enzymes, usually in the liver, to vitamin D3 (cholecalciferol) and by the kidneys to its most active form, vitamin D4 (Calcitriol). Calcitriol is a prescription drug use in people with renal failure.

With the pill supplements of vitamin D, I now see the pendulum swinging to the other side. Our society was previously very low on vitamin D, but now we are at risk of going to the other extreme. We need to find the proper balance, which resides in the middle.

Vitamin D forces our bodies to absorb calcium and phosphorous (NIH, ODS, 2020a). You may think that this is a good thing, but without the hormones in place to deposit the calcium and phosphate into the bones, the calcium and phosphate deposit into soft tissues (Bouillon, 2020). This is called metastatic calcification and the FDA warns that too much vitamin D can cause this (Bouillon, 2020). That is one reason why I do not routinely recommend calcium supplements to maintain strong bones (Siska, 2017). The first place we notice this calcification is in our kidneys, and it results in kidney failure (Black, 2003). This only happens in people who severely overdo taking vitamin D. See the chart below, which I formulated from data on National Institute of Health (NIH) websites for consumers. It is at the following link.

Dose of Vitamin D	Blood Levels that the Dose Usually Yields	What to Expect
10,000 to 40,000 IU/day	500–600 nmol/L (200–240 ng/mL).	Toxicities: absorption of too much calcium and phosphorous. Soft tissue calcification. Renal failure
10,000 IU/day to 6,000 IU/Day	125–150 nmol/L (50–60 ng/mL)	Possible toxicities listed above or listed below
5,000 I U/day	100–150 nmol/L (40–60 ng/mL), above 125 is the official danger zone	increases in all-cause mortality, greater risk of cancer at some sites like the pancreas, greater risk of cardiovascular events, and more falls and fractures among the elderly
Below 4,000 IU/day	75–120 nmol/L or 30–48 ng/mL	Bad things rarely happen in this range, but it is still possible.
The dose is variable but somewhere between 400 and 2,000 IU/day	≥50 nmol/L (≥20 ng/mL);	50 –75 nmol/L is the perfect serum level that covers the needs of 97.5% of the population.
	30–50 nmol/L (12–20 ng/mL).	Inadequate levels
	<30 nmol/L (<12 ng/mL)	This is considered a deficency:life is shortened, rickets in infants and children and osteomalacia in adults enerrgy levels are low, infections are common

This chart shows the pattern that most vitamins follow. When a vitamin deficiency is corrected and the vitamin level restored to normal, miraculous things happen. Life is extended, all diseases are made better, energy is restored, the immune system is optimized, chronic wounds heal, skin looks great, and mood is happy. There is no end to the goodness that a properly nourished body experiences.

But when a vitamin level already normal is elevated further with synthetic supplements, good things no longer happen; sometimes, bad things happen. In the case of vitamin D, renal failure may be the likely result of taking too much vitamin D for too long and not having blood levels monitored.

Rarely do we get too many vitamins from food. Also, it is impossible to get too much vitamin D from the sun.

Blood testing is key to attaining the optimal vitamin D level in our bodies and finding the perfect vitamin D dose for our individual needs. Until home monitoring blood tests are developed, we are dependent on doctors and laboratories to provide us with this information. That is why I recommend to my patients that they see a medical doctor if they suspect that they have a vitamin D deficiency.

People over 50 years of age are at high risk for vitamin deficiencies. As we age, our bodies can become less efficient at manufacturing and extracting precious vitamins and minerals from our food, so deficiencies can develop. Sometimes symptoms of deficiencies mimic signs of old age, and people resign themselves to living with them, supposing that these symptoms are inevitable. The same thing is also happening with vitamin B12 and magnesium

(Lundberg, 2015; McBride, 2000). People who live with these vitamin deficiencies often think that their symptoms are due to old age, even when they are not.

Not only do our bodies lose the ability to absorb these nutrients over time, but also common drugs deplete these nutrients from our bodies. Doctors can now test blood levels of B12 and see whether this deficiency is present. But magnesium is more complicated because it resides inside the cells. Only 1% of magnesium is in the bloodstream (where laboratories can test). Therefore, if a magnesium blood level is low, most likely a magnesium deficiency is causing the symptoms. However, often the magnesium blood levels are normal, but the patient has an undetected magnesium deficiency (Lundberg, 2015). (See Table 2.)

Table 2. Sneaky Deficiencies that Mimic Old Age

Essential Nutrient and Frequency of Deficiency	Drugs that Cause Deficiencies	Symptoms that Mimic Old Age	Symptoms that Are Never Normal
Vitamin D: 60% of nursing home residents and 57% of hospitalized patients were found to be vitamin D deficient (Tangpricha, 2016)	Dilantin, phenobarbital, and rifampin	Muscle weakness and pain, especially pressure applied to sternum or tibia; poor balance, frequent falls	Severely brittle bones; Hyperparathyroid disease (as the body desperately tries to compensate)
Vitamin B12 5-20% of those over 50 years are deficient. As many as 1 in 5 people over the age of 50. (McBride, 2000)	Alcoholic beverages; Glucophage (AKA metformin) a type 2 diabetes drug; drugs that treat heartburn and cause low stomach acid	Premature gray hair; blotchy skin; walking with feet far apart to keep balance; low energy, memory loss, brain fog	Anemia, with cells of an unusual size or shape; tingling in the hands, feet, arms, legs; unexplained weakness of the legs leading to paraplegia in extreme cases(13)
Magnesium: 75% of Americans don't consume enough magnesium and some experts say it is a nationwide deficiency. (7)	Alcoholic beverages; any drug that causes diarrhea; water pills (AKA diuretics)	Low energy, brain fog, muscle weakness, tremor, anxiety, apathy, irritability, depression, unstable walking	Abnormal eye movements called nystagmus, tetany, dizziness, seizures, delirium, and psychosis, abnormal heart beats

OVERT/OBVIOUS VITAMIN DEFICIENCIES

Overt vitamin deficiencies are obvious. Doctors usually diagnose them. Several vitamin deficiencies show up in the blood and skin. This occurs because skin and blood cells have a rapid turnover rate; they are constantly dying and being replaced. For example, a red blood cell only lives for three months. Our bodies are constantly building millions of blood cells and therefore need a constant supply of building material in the form of vitamins and minerals. The cells in the mouth, tongue surface, and lips also have a rapid turnover. Table 3 (below) lists a variety of signs of vitamin deficiency and the vitamins you should consider if you experience these signs.

Table 3. Signs of Vitamin Deficiency

If You Have:	You Could Have a Deficiency in:
Frequent nose bleeds, bleeding of the gums	vitamin C, vitamin K
Frequent colds and lung infections	Any vitamin or iron but especially Vitamins C, E, D and Zinc
Skin defects	vitamin C, A, B12, niacin, zinc
Defects in the mouth and tongue	vitamin C
Defects in hair	vitamin D, biotin, possibly others
Defects in nails	Too much zinc or too little calcium
Low energy	Any vitamin or iron, B vitamins, Magnesium,
Dry or irritated eyes, night blindness.	vitamin A or vitamin E
Chronic anemia without bleeding: The hallmark of poor intestinal absorption	Any vitamin, iron, folic acid, vitamin B12, vitamin C

UNBALANCED DIETS RESULT IN SINGLE VITAMIN DEFICIENCIES. MALABSORPTION RESULTS IN MULTIPLE VITAMIN DEFICIENCIES.

Water-soluble vitamin deficiencies were some of the first individual vitamin deficiencies to be detected. Hundreds of years ago, vitamin C and B deficiencies (especially thiamin and niacin) were common when most people's diets were poor and unbalanced. It became clear early on that people cannot live on bread alone. People must eat fruits and vegetables to be healthy. People with poor diets historically developed horrible diseases that shortened lives and often left otherwise young and healthy people deformed and disabled. But with slight changes to their diets, many people noticed that these problems went away. Let's look at how this happened for three diseases: scurvy, BeriBeri disease, and pellagra.

Sailors at sea for long periods whose diets lacked fruits and vegetables quickly developed scurvy. Early symptoms of scurvy include weakness, feeling tired, curly hair, and sore arms and legs. Without treatment, decreased red blood cells, gum disease, and bleeding from the skin may occur. As scurvy worsens, wounds don't heal well, people experience personality changes, and finally death results from infection or bleeding. What people discovered was that the symptoms went away quickly when fresh fruits and vegetables were added to their diet. Sailors on boats who ate lots of fruits and vegetables were able to avoid scurvy altogether.

BeriBeri is another example of a disease born solely from a vitamin deficiency. When people began processing brown rice into white rice for better taste and longer shelf life, those who ate only white rice suffered from nerve-related conditions, such as having decreased muscle function (particularly in the lower legs), tingling or loss of feeling in the feet and hands, pain, difficulty speaking, vomiting, involuntary eye movement, and even paralysis. In contrast, the people who ate brown rice did not experience these diseases. They stayed strong and healthy. When the brown husk was added back into the diets of the white-rice eaters, these nerve-related disorders went away. This led to the discovery of thiamin and the cure for the BeriBeri disease.

In the United States' South, about a century ago, there was an epidemic of skin lesions that looked similar to leprosy. These lesions were eventually traced back to a diet consisting predominantly of biscuits and corn. In 1915, a doctor named Joseph Goldberger was assigned to study this mystery disease by the surgeon general of the United States. Goldberger figured out that the skin lesions went away in people who ate bread made with a small amount of brewer's yeast. The yeast produced niacin, which cured pellagra, the mystery skin disease. Since then, niacin has been added to flour to prevent the disease of pellagra from recurring. Biscuits and gravy for everyone!

People who benefit from vitamins don't develop superhuman strength and abilities. They just become normal and equal to those who are properly nourished. For people healthy and well-nourished, vitamins are not going to do anything miraculous. Sometimes, good pills do bad things.

VITAMINS GET A BAD RAP BECAUSE PEOPLE DON'T USE THEM PROPERLY

At one time, healthy food was expensive, and nutritious diets were difficult to maintain. The U.S. Food and Drug Administration (FDA) set minimum dosages on specific vitamin and mineral intake for people to avoid diseases. Now that healthy food is plentiful and inexpensive common foods are fortified with vitamins, vitamin and mineral deficiencies are rare, so vitamin toxicities due to excessive consumption are a concern. The FDA has now set upper limits on intake for certain vitamins and minerals.

There are 31 essential nutrients that were evaluated by the FDA's advisors. Our bodies cannot make these chemicals, which are necessary for our biochemical reactions. We must obtain these essential nutrients from food or supplements to survive and avoid disease. However, there are exceptions. Our bodies make vitamin D from cholesterol in the skin when sunlight activates it. Also, the bacteria in our gut make vitamin K and B vitamins in minimal amounts. Of these 31 essential nutrients, 14 are vitamins; the rest, 17, are minerals. Half of the vitamins have maximum dosages not to be exceeded, according to the FDA. All 17 minerals have upper limits listed except arsenic, silicon, and chromium. It's already been established that most minerals should be consumed only in trace amounts.

Below is a list of the most common essential nutrients that have upper limits set by Nutrition Board, Institute of Medicine, National Academies. They are the advisors to the FDA. The National Academies are private nonprofit institutions that provide independent and objective analysis and advice to the FDA and conduct other activities to solve complex problems and inform public policy decisions related to science, technology, and medicine. The Academies operate under an 1863 congressional charter to the National Academy of Sciences, which was signed by President Lincoln. (See Table 4.)

Table 4. Dietary Reference Intakes (DRI): Tolerable Upper Intake Levels

Essential nutrient	Max dose for Adults Without Special Needs	Effects When Levels Go Too High	Personal Thoughts on Synthetic Pills Only (*Not applicable to food sources.*)
Vitamin A	3,000 µg/d	Teratological effects, liver toxicity	The FDA minimized the problems with vitamin A orally. Only eye doctors, oncologists, and dermatologists should be recommending this vitamin. It's great topically for amazing skin.
Vitamin D	4,000 IU/d (the maximum daily allowance for those older than 71 yrs old is 800 IU/d)	Hypercalcemia can lead to decreased renal function and hypercalciuria, kidney failure, cardiovascular system failure, and calcification of soft tissues	Normalizing this deficiency will extend life, increase energy levels, reduce the occurrence of infection improve any disease state. Renal/cardiovascular consequences are serious. It causes too much calcium and phosphate absorption. Monitoring blood levels is key! Home monitoring blood kits are needed.
Vitamin E	1,000 mg/d	Hemorrhagic toxicity	There are more concerns not mentioned here. It's best when used topically for great skin.
Niacin	35 mg/d	Flushing and gastrointestinal distress	It's useless for cardiovascular disease, but a good pre-workout supplement due to its role making ATP.
Vitamin B6 /pyridoxine	100 mg/d	Sensory neuropathy	Symptom severity appears to be dose-dependent; symptoms stop when it is discontinued.
Folate	1,000 µg/d	Masks neurological complication in people with vitamin B12 deficiency. Applies to synthetic forms	Too much can cause cancer, and not enough can also cause cancer. Food sources deliver the perfect amount.
Vitamin C	2,000 mg/d	GI disturbances, kidney stones, excess iron absorption	It's one of the first vitamins to get depleted in times of physical stress, dehydration, famine, exposure to toxins, etc. Our skin loves this vitamin.
Choline	3,500 mg/d	Fishy body odor, sweating, salivation, hypotension, hepatotoxicity	It is on the FDA vitamin list with upper limits, so I mentioned it. (No one ever asks me about this vitamin.)
Calcium	2000 mg/d 2,500 mg/d for 31– 50-year-old females	Kidney stones, hypercalcemia, hypercalciuria, prostate cancer, constipation, soft tissue calcification	You need hormones to put the calcium in your bones. Do not take this in excess with excess vitamin D. Soft tissue calcification and metastatic calcification mean that you are turning into a stone statue. See phosphorous.
Phosphorous	4,000 mg/d	Metastatic calcification, skeletal porosity with calcium absorption	Fitness gurus use this because it's part of ATP and energy production. Food sources are safest. The side effects form pills/powders are very serious.
Selenium	400 µg/d	Hair and nail brittleness and loss	Hair loss is a mysterious and upsetting effect

Source: Institute of Medicine, National Academies. (n.d.).

Vitamins and minerals are natural, but they are not always safe in unnatural doses from synthetic forms. The goal is to have vitamin levels in the healthy zone. Just as with food, water, oxygen, or sunshine, too much or too little has adverse effects. In the hospital, we measure calcium, sodium, potassium, phosphate, chloride, and magnesium. All these natural elements need to be in the natural zone; otherwise, bad things happen.

THE DOSE ON THE VITAMIN BOTTLE MEANS ABSOLUTELY NOTHING!

There are four types of dosages, depending on the situation and goal of treatment. To maintain this optimal range, the National Institutes of Health put upper and lower limits on certain vitamins. The **lower limit** is the dose needed to prevent a disease. **Upper limit** dosages are not to be exceeded, or you can develop toxic side effects. **Treatment doses** are to be determined by a medical doctor based on the severity of the disease and dosing guidelines.

A **therapeutic dose** is when a high dose is used for a **short period to time** to achieve a therapeutic effect, much as with a drug. This is a rare occurrence that only is possible with a few vitamins and minerals. It happens with magnesium, vitamin c, and zinc. This is an evolving area of medicine. Lots of studies and experiments are being conducted to reevaluate more products and more therapeutic effects.

Magnesium is used as a muscle relaxer at high doses. High doses of Zinc and Vitamin C are used as adjuvants to chemotherapy regimens.

WHICH MEDICAL EXPERTS DECIDE ON THE DOSAGES AND OTHER GUIDELINES?

The FDA, Institute of Medicine, National Academies, Nutrition Board, and the U.S. Task Force are some of the government agencies that make up the National Institutes of Health. They are all government agencies, and they all stick together on their statements. They have no financial motive (e.g., they have no conflict of interest). If anything, their motive seems to be to prevent consumer fraud and consumer deception. They are very concerned about manufacturers and sellers of dietary supplements who make exaggerated claims about natural supplements to profit financially at the expense of the consumers.

BACK TO THE BEGINNING

So let's reexamine two opposing commonly voiced opinions from this chapter's beginning: "Vitamins are a waste of money" and "Healthy people don't need vitamins to stay healthy." These statements are generally true, except for healthy people who are under a lot of physical stress and/or are at risk of washing out their water-soluble vitamins. This is the case for marathon runners, smokers, people who drink alcohol, and people who take prescription drugs.

Another claim from the beginning of the chapter:

"You can prevent certain cancers and cardiovascular disease with specific supplements regardless of your health." This is also true, but only if you have a vitamin deficiency and you restore it to normal. Only then will the cancer and heart attack risks decrease. However, if you are already in the perfect vitamin zone and in a peak state of nutrition, vitamins are not going to prevent cancer or heart disease, and consuming vitamin supplements might even cause or accelerate those diseases in certain individuals. Both sides are right and wrong. The truth lies somewhere in the middle—in the gray area.

3

CORRECTING EXCESSIVE OXIDATIVE DAMAGE

WHAT IS AN ANTIOXIDANT?

Have you ever seen hydrogen peroxide poured onto an open wound? The liquid forms bubbles as it consumes the dead, infected flesh. The right amount cleans up the wound. However, if the hydrogen peroxide solution is too strong, damage to healthy tissue takes place. Antioxidants stop that from happening inside our body.

Antioxidants stop excessive oxidative damage by inactivating rogue fly-away electrons and other molecular parts. Otherwise, these unstable particles can get loose and dissolve everything in their path. Free radicals destroy cell membranes, receptors, and enzymes. Too much free radical activity causes inflammation. Therefore, a little bit of natural hydrogen peroxide is good and natural, but too much is harmful.

Oxygen is thought to be the most common free radical in the body—yes, the good old-fashioned oxygen that we breathe. Have you ever noticed how lettuce and other delicate vegetables are preserved and stay fresh longer when put into an airtight container to reduce exposure to oxygen? More potent than the oxygen that we breathe are oxygen-containing molecules such as hydrogen peroxide and hypochlorous acid, which can change into the super strong radical anions (negatively charged ions) called hydroxyl (-OH) and other destructive anions.

Some people drink hydrogen peroxide in the belief that this will improve their health. They then take antioxidant pills. For those people, I say: Stop micromanaging your body. It knows what to do. Our bodies are smarter than we are. A healthy body produces the perfect amount of internal free radicals.

WHICH VITAMINS, MINERALS, NUTRACEUTICALS, AND HERBS HAVE ANTIOXIDANT PROPERTIES?

One of the main tests is called the oxygen radical absorbance capacity (ORAC). Other measurement tests include the Folin-Ciocalteu reagent and the trolox equivalent antioxidant capacity assay. According to the Natural Medicine Database (2020), the following products have noticeable antioxidant activity: selenium (Se), strawberry (Fragaria spp.), black currant (Ribes nigrum), blackberry (Rubus fructicosus), carrot (Daucus carota), cranberry (Vaccinium macrocarpon), dandelion (Taraxacum officinale), globe artichoke (Cynara scolymus L.), lutein, lycopene, melatonin, noni (Morinda citrifolia), pycnogenol (Pinus pinaster ssp. atlantica), raspberry (Rubus idaeus), seaweed/kelp/bladderwrack (Fucus vesiculosus), vitamin A (retinol), vitamin E and vitamin C.

MELATONIN, AN UNLIKELY ANTIOXIDANT?

Melatonin supplements are used to help induce sleep because it is released naturally by the pineal gland in the brain and helps us fall asleep at night when it is dark. Melatonin is very connected with our circadian rhythm and the environment. Recently, it was discovered that melatonin's endocrine properties extend to the skin and hair. Could that be why animals shed their fur in the summer and grow thicker fur in the winter? Perhaps. We do know that there are melatonin receptors in the skin and hair follicles (Kleszczynski & Fischer, 2012). Our skin makes the melatonin that is needed to keep our skin healthy and youthful. Taking melatonin orally does not have the same effect, so people may see a surfeit of topical melatonin products. Melatonin keeps our skin healthy and youthful by two major mechanisms. It has antioxidant effects that neutralize the oxidative damage from the sun, and it stimulates growth receptors in the skin. The antioxidant effects of melatonin are so strong that they are thought to be more potent than glutathione (López-Burillo et al., 2003), vitamin C (Montilla-Lopez et al., 2002), and vitamin E (Mayo et al., 2003). Melatonin is also being studied in other areas of health, such as neurodegenerative diseases, cancers, and antiaging.

ANTIOXIDANTS AND ATHLETES

Unfortunately, emerging evidence indicates that antioxidant use can impede athletic performance in healthy individuals. A 2015 article (Braakhuis & Hopkins, 2015) looked at the use of vitamin E, quercetin, resveratrol, beetroot juice, other food-derived polyphenols, spirulina, and N-acetylcysteine (NAC) in athletes. The authors concluded that acute intake of Vitamin E and NAC is likely to be beneficial. However, chronic intake of most other antioxidants has harmful effect on performance (Braakhuis & Hopkins, 2015). The Academy of Nutrition and Dietetics, Dietitians of Canada and the American College of Sports Medicine supported this conclusion and do not recommend the use of antioxidants to counteract the oxidative stress from exercise (Frijhoff et al., 2015; Position, 2016).

Perhaps a healthy body really does take the perfect approach to free radicals. This reinforces my belief that natural is best and that our bodies are smarter than we are. Despite this negative information, I believe that antioxidant pills do have their place in therapy. They must be used wisely like drugs and medicine to bring an unhealthy body back into alignment with natural health.

USING ANTIOXIDANT PILLS TO TREAT CERTAIN DISEASE STATES

The Food and Drug Administration (FDA) says we should never use dietary supplements to treat a disease. If a person has a disease that is progressing and can potentially shorten a person's life, that person is advised to see a medical professional for evidence-based treatments and monitoring of the condition. However, there is emerging evidence that antioxidants can be used to improve, but not halt, certain disease states that involve high oxidative stress. Diabetes is one such example.

ANTIOXIDANTS FOR DIABETICS

Researchers have reported that diabetics have increased blood concentrations of the byproduct from lipid peroxidation called thiobarbituric acid reactive substances (Balbi et al., 2018). The presence of these substances in high amounts is a marker of excessive free radicals that lead to damage to cell membranes and potential critically important bioactive proteins. It is thought that antioxidants can intervene and bring the body back into a more natural state with less oxidative stress.

The journal *Diabetology & Metabolic Syndrome* published a systematic review and meta-analysis that looked at 12 randomized control trials to see the effects of vitamins B, C, D, and E in type 2 diabetics (Ametov et al., 2003). The researchers concluded that using vitamin E may be a valuable strategy for controlling complications from diabetes and enhancing antioxidant capacity. Vitamin E is oil-soluble and has a strong affinity for cell membranes, which are mainly made up of lipids and fats. Vitamin E is also used in grocery stores to keep raw meat looking fresh by preventing it from turning a grayish brown when exposed to air. Vitamin E is also used in fish oils to prevent the oil from turning rancid. Therefore, it was no surprise that it performed well in this meta-analysis.

To a lesser degree, vitamin C also performed well. It is water-soluble and goes where vitamin E cannot, as oil and water do not mix. Vitamin C is known for keeping freshly cut fruit from becoming discolored when exposed to air.

The meta-analysis briefly mentioned good results from glutathione, a water-soluble antioxidant that many people believe is the most potent antioxidant that our body makes. It's currently being used in hospitals to counteract the negative effects of excessive Tylenol consumption and during other times of exposure to toxins.

Unfortunately, the meta-analysis did not mention Alpha-lipoic acid (ALA). ALA is another potent antioxidant that our bodies make, one that is used in hospitals to counteract the nerve toxicities from chemotherapy. It is soluble in water and oil and therefore can go anywhere in the body. Diabetics have used ALA, and they stated in the Sidney 1 and 2 Trials that they could feel it working (Ziegler et al., 2006). Up to 62 percent of the 181 patients in the Sidney 2 Trial treated with ALA perceived a greater than 50 percent reduction in neuropathic symptoms (Pérez-Sánchez et al., 2018, p. 403). The ALA-treated group felt an improvement in the stabbing pain, burning pain, paresthesia, and asleep numbness (Pérez-Sánchez et al., 2018, p. 403).

ANTIOXIDANTS FOR THE SKIN

What about antioxidants for the skin? Could they improve the appearance of wrinkles or possibly prevent the formation of wrinkles? Vitamin A and C, as well as melatonin, have antioxidant properties and also have receptor activities in the skin that help stimulate collagen growth and repair. Vitamin C also has activities within the melanin and skin pigment system with mild skin lightening activities. Vitamin E is also a powerful antioxidant for the skin, but I'm unaware of any receptor activity.

Vitamin C and Vitamin E pills consumed together orally have been shown in several medical studies to protect the skin from the harmful effects of the sun and to prevent sunburn. They do not absorb the UVA or UVB spectrum radiation, so they are not sunscreens, but they do neutralize the oxidative damage cause by the UV light. These pills protect the skin from the sun and reduce the severity of the sunburn that otherwise would occur (Pérez-Sánchez et al., 2018, p. 403).

Vitamin A, carotenoids, coenzyme Q10, and melatonin are all antioxidants that are being used for the skin. However, Vitamin A, Vitamin C, and melatonin also play a role in collagen and elastin production (Pérez-Sánchez et al., 2018, p. 403). All these antioxidants are being used both topically and orally ((Pérez-Sánchez et al., 2018, p. 403).

ANTIOXIDANTS FOR THE EYES

Occasionally, eye doctors will prescribe oral antioxidants for specific eye conditions. In addition to that, Vitamin A deficiency can lead to blindness. Supplementation is used in this case, although not for its antioxidant activities. Vitamin C, vitamin E, and beta-carotene, and zinc reduced the risk of developing the advanced stage of age-related macular degeneration by 25 percent in people who had the intermediate stage of this disease or who had the advanced stage in only one eye (National Eye Institute, 2020). In another study, adding lutein and zeaxanthin (two carotenoids found in the eye) improved the supplements' effectiveness in people who were not taking beta-carotene and those who consumed only small amounts of lutein and zeaxanthin in foods (National Eye Institute, 2020).

ANTIOXIDANTS FOR THE LUNGS

Antioxidants are used in a nebulized inhaled form to treat cystic fibrosis and other lung diseases. The antioxidant in question is called N-acetylcysteine. It mitigates the oxidative damage and thins mucus to preserve lung function (Sadowska et al., 2006). However, when Vitamin E was added to e-cigarette vaping formulations to help preserve lung function, it backfired. Instead, Vitamin E administered in that way caused lung damage. To understand this, we must recognize that Vitamin E is a collective term used to describe eight different natural compounds. These compounds are called tocopherol and tocotrienol and they are subclassified as alpha, beta, gamma, and delta (Stanner et al., 2004).

Synthetic vitamin E pills usually contain only one of these eight compounds, alpha-tocopherol. It's very unnatural for a single antioxidant to be found in nature or in our body alone and in high amounts. Antioxidants need each other to function properly (Rizvi et al., 2014). They need to juggle electrons between themselves to perform their antioxidant activities. After they absorb rogue flay-way electrons, they toss their unwanted electrons to a different antioxidant that needs electrons to execute its necessary functions. This juggling enables both antioxidants to return to their original state and repeat the process of neutralizing excessive free radicals. This is called synergy, and it is demonstrated in many studies (Pullar et al., 2017; Rizvi et al., 2014).

Vitamin E and C especially have good synergy together. This has been tested both orally and topically. Researches saw the ability of these compounds to neutralize the oxidative damage caused from the sun in people with fair skin. Researchers could measure the redness caused when the vitamins were used alone and together (Pullar et al., 2017).

Going back to synthetic vitamin E being inhaled and applied topically to lung tissue, this is what went wrong: The single tocotrienol did not have another antioxidant in high amounts to juggle electrons back and forth with. It is my opinion that vitamin E in the vaping formulations got what it needed in terms of electrons from the surrounding lung tissue. That is how the damage occurred. This was similar to inhaling battery acid, which is why young healthy people started showing up in the emergency rooms coughing up blood and ending up in respiratory failure as a result of vaping (Agustin et al., 2018).

ANTIOXIDANTS FOR THE HEART

Smoking, excessive alcohol intake, and illicit drug use can lead to heart damage in people as young as in their thirties. Biomarkers prove that the oxidative damage affects the heart muscles (Balbi et al., 2018). Some people swear that antioxidants have slowed or halted their heart disease. It is possible that there are genetic variations and mutations in these individuals' biochemistry, especially involving vitamin C (He et al., 2017).

Bad health is a downward spiral, and sometimes it is accelerated by oxidative stress, especially from excessive smoking and alcohol intake. Researchers are working diligently to understand how they can intervene effectively and reliably. But until they do, we must intervene through prudent lifestyle choices.

4

OPTIMIZING THE GUT

Many doctors believe that healing the gut is essential to healing the body. How could this one organ have such a profound effect on the entire body?

SIX WAYS THE GUT CAN MAKE OR BREAK YOUR HEALTH

1. Biochemical reactions take place here.
2. The immune system is located here.
3. Leaky gut contributes to systemic inflammation.
4. Latent infections or dysbiosis can occur here.
5. Removal of toxins and waste occur here.
6. Nutrients are extracted here. (See Table 5.)

Table 5. Six Ways the Gut can Affect Our Health

How the gut affects health	How this happens	Natural products that help
Biochemical reactions	Vitamin K, and B vitamins are made here. Anti-inflammatory compounds are made here. Compounds to protect from colon cancer. Other toxins can be broken down here.	Probiotics and prebiotics are being studied to do the job of the liver and the kidneys in times of organ failure. Saccharomyces is a probiotic that makes niacin vitamin B
The immune system	The gut is headquarters for the WBC's. They "sample" the contents in the gut and make antibodies when needed.	Probiotics: See chart for products on the market. Glutamate (other amino acids) can also strengthen the immune system.
Leaky gut	A damaged gut leaks toxins into the bloodstream and causes systemic inflammation.	Fasting and whole foods are key. Probiotics? Prebiotics? Glutamate, possibly other amino acids.
Infections	To remove bad bacteria: H. Pylori, c-diff, MRSA, fungus, and other uninvited pathogens can live here and sabotage our health.	Probiotics are nature's antibiotics. They can decolonize and help fight off bad bacteria, such as c-diff, MRSA, and H-pylori
Removal of toxic waste	Probiotics for diarrhea. Fiber for daily bowel movements or to firm up the stool and alleviate diarrhea. Constipation: Magnesium.	Magnesium pills are best to mitigate the horrible taste of liquid formulations. Milk of Magnesia and Epson salt are low-cost options.
Extracting nutrients	A healthy intestinal lining is necessary.	Digestive enzymes, pancrealipase(Rx), and other natural products

A HEALTHY GUT MAKES BIOCHEMICALS AND VITAMINS

Biochemical reactions take place in the gut, as if the gut were a type of miniature liver. These reactions include detoxifying and eliminating. Also, the manufacturing of B vitamins, vitamin K, and possibly other necessary biochemicals occurs in the gut. Researchers are discovering that our gut and the bacteria that live makes the gut another organ similar to a liver that performs biochemical reactions. The gut bacteria make vitamins, break down toxins, make neurochemicals that affect our brain and mood, and make anti-inflammatory molecules that can protect against colon cancer.

The bacteria in our gut are involved in producing B vitamins, such as pantothenic acid (B5), pyridoxine (B6), riboflavin (B2), thiamine (B1), vitamin B12, and vitamin K. These bacteria don't make enough to help us thrive and achieve high levels of such vitamins; quite the contrary. They only make enough to keep us alive. They don't even make enough to sustain a healthy pregnancy when there is a lack of fruits and veggies in the pregnant woman's diet. (Hill, 1997).

This minimal level of vitamin production in the gut became apparent when the pellagra outbreak occurred in the southern part of the United Stated in the early 1900s. Pellagra is an overt dietary deficiency of vitamin B3, niacin. By 1926, a medical doctor had established that a diet of foods high in niacin or a small amount of brewer's yeast prevented pellagra. Brewer's yeast or baker's yeast is another name for the probiotic Saccharomyces. Saccharomyces manufactures niacin in the gut (Swan, 2005).

A healthy gut breaks down toxins and makes healthy biochemicals. Healthy bacteria also make anti-inflammatory chemicals and other chemicals that strengthen the barrier of the gut to keep toxins in the lumen of the gut and out of the bloodstream. A healthy gut also produces the neurochemicals involved in brain function and emotions. More on this subject in the detox chapter and the mind/body chapter.

LATENT INFECTION AND DYSBIOSIS OF THE GUT CAN SABOTAGE GOOD HEALTH

An unhealthy gut is also a source of inflammation when bad bacteria and yeasts or fungus grow out of control. H. Pylori, MRSA, and C-diff are common infections of the gastro-intestinal (GI) tract that cause havoc throughout the body and possibly trigger auto-immune diseases, as in the case of H. Pylori and Hashimoto's disease or rosacea. Epidemiologic studies report a higher prevalence of Helicobacter Pylori (*H. Pylori*) infection in the elderly, with a ratio of over 70% in patients with gastrointestinal diseases and approximately 60% in asymptomatic patients (Cizginer et al., 2014). With regards to MRSA, in 2018, the Food and Drug Administration (FDA) sent out a press release that acknowledged that MRSA colonizes the gut and then causes recurrent infections throughout the body. The FDA also stated that a specific probiotic of the Subtills species can decolonize MRSA from the GI tract (NIH, 2018).

C-diff is a form of infectious diarrhea. It is highly contagious and difficult to eradicate because it produces hard to penetrate spores. It also leaves behind toxins that unleash havoc in the body.

NATURAL DIGESTIVE ENZYMES: EXTRACTING NUTRIENTS

The lining of the gut must be healthy and free of inflammation and disease. These intestinal cells in our intestines are like shoppers that take the perfect amount of nutrients from the gut and move it into the bloodstream for the body's use. That is how food delivers the perfect amount of vitamins and minerals to keep us in the perfect zone.

Pancrealipase is a prescription product to help people with cystic fibrosis and other conditions to dissolve and digest their food. Without these products, cystic fibrosis patients have bloating, abdominal pain, diarrhea, constipation, and other unpleasant symptoms. Natural digestive enzymes can be found in whole foods, such as pineapple, mango, papaya, kefir, bananas, avocados, and sauerkraut. Additionally, natural products exist in pill form for this indication.

HEALING A DAMAGED GUT WITH AMINO ACIDS

The contents of the intestines can leak out into the surrounding tissues and cause systemic inflammation. Fasting and eating whole foods and curing any underlying diseases will do the most benefit to heal and correct a leaky gut, but what about other natural products such as glutamate and other amino acids?

Glutamate is an amino acid that many people take to heal the gut. Studies show that it promotes intestinal mucosal cell growth and repair in patients who are receiving chemotherapy and radiotherapy, both of which cause intestinal mucosal damage, such as stomatitis and mucositis. Glutamate is also being studied in leaky gut to reduce intestinal permeability and bacterial translocation. Additionally, several studies have shown that glutamine has a positive effect on the immune response. Glutamine supplementation decreased bacterial colonization and promoted the activation of innate and adaptive immunity (Perna et al., 2019). Many products on the market strengthen the immune system by strengthening other parts of the body. Glutamate is one such product.

THE IMPORTANCE OF DAILY BOWEL MOVEMENTS

Our intestines are how our body eliminates wastes and toxins. Constipation is an uncomfortable yet common problem that can get worse with age, but for anyone with this condition, I say, CONGRATULATIONS! You now qualify for my favorite natural product that can cause diarrhea in many people. I'm taking about magnesium, the active ingredient in milk of magnesia (MOM).

Magnesium has many health benefits. It plays an essential role in more than 300 cellular reactions, including the formation of energy (Shils et al., 1994). You might also recall from chapter two that it is a pervasive and insidious vitamin deficiency. I recommend magnesium oxide 400-mg pills: 1–2 pills, 1–2 times a day, as needed, to produce daily bowel movements. Excess magnesium is eliminated through the kidneys, so it is difficult to get too much of it unless you have kidney failure. Those people should not be taking any extra vitamins or minerals without their doctors' consent.

Many people take magnesium at night before going to bed because it can cause drowsiness. It is also known as the relaxation mineral

CHRONIC DIARRHEA

Chronic diarrhea is a symptom that something else is wrong. If left untreated, it can lead to malabsorption of nutrients, vitamin deficiencies, and a downward spiral of bad health. Sometimes diarrhea can be treated with probiotics and fiber to firm up the stool. The best indication for probiotics is diarrhea. If you want to "wow" and impress your friends with your pharmaceutical knowledge, just recommend probiotics for diarrhea that is not associated with bowel disease. Under these conditions, probiotics work wonders. Probiotics treat diarrhea by keeping bad bacteria in check, by producing biochemicals that are astringent in action, by producing anti-inflammatory chemicals, and by many more mechanisms of actions that are still being discovered.

PROBIOTIC FOR THE IMMUNE SYSTEM

The gut comprises 70–80% of the immune system. Consider the gut as the headquarters for the immune system (Vighi et al., 2008). Our intestinal cells sample the bacteria in our gut and provide information to our immune system to help it develop better and become stronger. I was fascinated to see that Bifidobacterium *longum BB536* was given as an adjunct to the flu vaccine (Namba et al., 2010). I think that this was brilliant, considering that often, vaccines don't work because the person's immune system is too weak and debilitated to mount a response and make the necessary immunological ammunition.

For severely immune-compromised patients, I don't recommend probiotics. Probiotics are live bacteria that can in rare cases cause an infection and sepsis. This can occur to premature babies, cancer patients, and anyone else in a fragile and debilitated state (Boyle et al., 2006). Probiotics are very dose-dependent and they are also live bacteria/fungus, so I don't recommend soon-to-expire probiotics that are on sale. I also do not recommend frozen yogurt or frozen kefir because the freezing will destroy and inactivate the medicinal properties of the product.

Technically, pill forms of probiotics are freeze-dried in a laboratory; adding moisture will bring them back to life. Storage, dose, and expiration date are all important. Packages have specific instructions from the manufacture that should be followed to ensure that the live organisms reach the site of action in the proper dose.

PROBIOTICS FOR OTHER CONDITIONS

Seasonal allergies, cholesterol, dental caries, women's health and infections, acne, eczema, weight loss and weight gain. Some bacteria and probiotics are also involved in the protection of colon cancer, specifically bifidobactia.

CHOOSING THE RIGHT PROBIOTIC FOR THE RIGHT PURPOSE

Probiotics are a subset of medicine. They are as individual as the various pharmacological drugs on the market. They have different indications and mechanisms of action. A probiotic database can help you find the right probiotic for the right purpose. My favorite free probiotic database is AEProbio, but there are others such as Medline Plus.

ConsumerLabs.com and NaturalMedicines.TherapeuticResearch.com are also good databases, but they require a subscription fee.

THE FUTURE OF PROBIOTICS AND PREBIOTICS

The possibilities for probiotics are endless, especially when you add prebiotics to the mix. Prebiotics either provide the building blocks for the chemical reaction or they provide the food to fuel the probiotic and give it energy so that it can perform the chemical reaction. There is research to support the thesis that the longevity gene is activated with probiotics, specifically with B. subtilis (yes, the same probiotic that decolonizes and kills MRSA). This probiotic has the ability to down-regulate the insulin-like signaling system that is essential in the healthy longevity of human centenarians. Could B. subtilis be incorporated into foods and beverages to extend human life expectancy and stop the development of age-related diseases (Ayala et al., 2017)?

CONCLUSION

Gut health is a hot topic, with new information coming in every day. Yes, a healthy gut is needed to have a healthy body, good energy, and good mood. But it is only one piece to the puzzle. Probiotics and prebiotics are an exciting area of new development and possibilities.

5

REDUCING INFLAMMATION WITH NATURAL PRODUCTS

There are several types of inflammation: acute, chronic, systemic, and localized. Acute and localized is when you get injured, and the inflammatory processes bring in the repair cells to heal the injury. An example would be a sprained ankle. If the injury does not heal quickly, then it becomes chronic and localized. An example of that would be a back injury or a neck injury.

Systemic and chronic is the type that we live with but don't really know that it's there. It slowly creeps up on us over time. It's everywhere and nowhere in particular. It's puffy eyes, stiff achy joints, and irritability. Many experts believe that this type of inflammation accelerates certain disease states, such as Alzheimer's disease, Parkinson's disease, multiple sclerosis, epilepsy, cerebral injury, cardiovascular disease, metabolic syndrome, cancer, allergies, asthma, bronchitis, colitis, arthritis, renal ischemia, psoriasis, diabetes, obesity, depression, fatigue, and acquired immune deficiency syndrome (AIDS) (Khansari et al., 2009; López-Otín et al., 2013; Roma & Jailal, 2018).

WHAT MEDICAL EXPERTS SAY ABOUT DISEASES OF AGING AND INFLAMMATION

The American Heart Association (2020) stated on its website that more information is needed on this subject and statin drugs work partially by reducing inflammation within the blood vessel walls. Current research includes a Cardiovascular Inflammation Reduction Trial (CIRT) and a Canakinumab Anti-Inflammatory Thrombosis Outcomes Study (CANTOS) trial involving canakinumab, an interleukin (IL)-1β neutralizing monoclonal antibody. These trials are in the process of validating inflammation as a viable target for preventing cardiovascular disease. Preliminary results show that there is a link, and possible interventions (Ridker, 2019).

The National Cancer Institute/National Institutes of Health (2020) stated on its website that over time, chronic inflammation can cause DNA damage and lead to cancer. People with chronic inflammatory bowel diseases, such as ulcerative colitis and Crohn's disease, have an increased risk of colon cancer.

The American Diabetes Association has not issued an official statement regarding diabetes and its link to inflammation. However, in a press release (American Diabetes Association, 2019), it mentioned that salsalate (an anti-inflammatory drug) improves diabetes.

OTHER INTERVENTIONS TO REDUCE SYSTEMIC INFLAMMATION

The following table list areas to explore for possible intervention. (See Table 6.)

Table 6. Other Interventions to Reduce Systemic Inflammation

Intervention to reduce inflammation	Causes of inflammation	Google search terms
Fasting and calorie restriction	leaky gut and over-nutrition	Intermittent fasting, leaky gut, chronic systemic inflammation, over-nutrition, obesity and inflammation.
The Paleo Diet	Removal of food allergens	Paleo diet, food allergens, and systemic inflammation
Impeccable oral and dental care	The link between gum disease and inflammation	periodontal disease, systemic inflammation, and the risk of cardiovascular disease
Avoid toxins	Excessive alcohol, smoke, illicit drug use, excessive sun exposure	Excessive alcohol consumption, inflammation, smoking, illicit drug use and inflammation
Hidden infections, sometimes called latent infections, dysbiosis in the gut, or chronic infections	Hidden bacteria, fungus, virus, and parasites can cause inflammation.	Inflammation and chronic infections, latent infections, dysbiosis in the gut, chronic strep throat and inflammation, candidiasis and inflammation
Post-infection syndrome	Bacteria can leave behind toxins, or viruses and other pathogens can cause a post-infection syndrome.	This is an emerging area of medicine.

CAN WE INTERVENE WITH NATURAL PRODUCTS?

Yes, we can intervene with diet, natural products, and a change in lifestyle. But as far as natural supplements are concerned, the two most talked-about supplements are omega-3 oils and turmeric. Other less known options are Morinda (Noni) juice, Bromelain (Ananas comosus), cat's claw (Uncaria guianensis), devil's claw (Harpagophytum procumbens), stinging nettle (Urtica dioica), and willow bark (Salix species).

HOW OMEGA-3S AND OTHER MEDICINAL OILS CALM INFLAMMATION

Omega-3s are active ingredients in medicinal oils: fish oils, flaxseed oil, olive oil, and a few other oils. These oils can be purchased in pill form or in a culinary form for cooking and making salads (Proudman & Cleland, 2010). The NIH (2020) website listed all the foods and oils high in omega-3s. It does not list olive oil, but some manufactures list the omega-3 content in their olive oil. Also, the Mediterranean diet, which includes olive oil as a staple, has amazing health and longevity effects. Therefore, many people consider olive oil to be a medicinal oil, even though it doesn't have high levels of omega-3s.

Omega-3s and other healthy oils are the building blocks of cell membranes. When a healthy cell becomes damaged, the torn cell membrane becomes the chemical signal to bring in the repair crew. The repair crew has white blood cells and the inflammatory mediators. For an acute injury, the inflammatory mediators resolve the problems and facilitate the repairs. However, for chronic inflammation, the inflammatory mediators just cause havoc, as there is nothing to fix.

Medicinal oils are very similar in chemical structure to the inflammatory signalers. Other names for omega-3s include EPA and DHA. These molecules can compete with arachidonic acid (an inflammatory chemical) for enzymes. Therefore, higher concentrations of EPA and DHA than arachidonic acid tip the eicosanoid balance toward less inflammatory activity (Proudman & Cleland, 2010).

However, widespread inflammation and swelling can be quite complicated. There are many signaling biochemicals, two of which are interleukins and tumor necrosis factor. When systemic inflammation is out of control, all these chemicals need to be dealt with. It appears that Omega-3 oils can help a little, but not enough to change a bad outcome.

HOW TURMERIC CALMS INFLAMMATION

Turmeric, also known as curcumin, is a root spice similar to ginger. It is an ancient herb that has been used for centuries in India and elsewhere in Asia for medicinal properties and promoting longevity. According to naturaldatabase.com, the best evidence supports its use in treating arthritis (rheumatoid and osteo), hay fever-type allergies, ulcerative colitis, depression, hyperlipidemia, nonalcoholic fatty liver disease, and itching. However, turmeric must be consumed for weeks before the beneficial effects are noticed. It does not work immediately, as we generally expect of over-the-counter medications such as ibuprofen.

According to Natural Medicines (2020), curcumin, the active ingredient in turmeric, seems to produce anti-inflammatory activity, possibly by inhibiting cyclooxygenase-2 (COX-2), prostaglandins, leukotrienes, tumor necrosis factor, and other cytokines involved in pro-inflammatory signaling pathways. Natural Medicines (2020) listed 10 different references to support this statement. It also reported that curcumin also seems to inhibit inflammatory enzymes such as collagenase, elastase, and hyaluronidase. Inflammation and infections often go hand in hand. It is no wonder that turmeric is being studied for possible antiviral effects with the Covid-19 virus and other viruses (Khaerunnis et al., 2020; Mounce et al., 2017).

TURMERIC AS A PAIN PILL

Anti-inflammatory drugs, such as ibuprofen and prednisone, double as pain medications. Natural products that reduce inflammation can also treat and alleviate pain. However, the onset of actions from natural supplements is subtler. Natural supplements could take days or weeks to start working. For people living with chronic pain who are desperate for relief, natural supplements, especially turmeric, offer hope.

Long-term and consistent use of these products is crucial.

In a 2016 evaluation of the medical literature (a meta-analysis), turmeric was compared with ibuprofen and diclofenac. The results showed that 8 to 12 weeks of standardized turmeric extracts, typically 1000 mg/day of curcumin, resulted in pain relief and reduction of inflammation similar to the benefits of anti-inflammatory drugs ibuprofen and diclofenac. The study evaluated people with various types of arthritis, including osteo arthritis and rheumatoid arthritis (Daily et al., 2016). Unfortunately, omega-3 oils didn't seem to affect pain. Their role seems to be more of an immune stabilizer with regards to systemic inflammation.

HOW SAFE ARE THESE NATURAL PRODUCTS?

Turmeric as a food source seems to be very safe; however, when taken in high doses (8,000 mg–12,000 mg) in a pill form, there is a potential for mild nausea and diarrhea (Daily et al., 2016). Also, there is a concern that high doses of turmeric could alter the metabolism of other drugs. There is a case report of a 54-year-old man who took about 15 spoonfuls of turmeric every day for 10 days. That is equivalent to 1,000 mg three times a day. In general, 1 tsp yields 200 mg of curcumin, depending on the product

(Natural Medicine, 2020). He was on tacrolimus to prevent kidney rejection after a transplant. The turmeric altered the enzymes in his liver, and this alteration caused toxic accumulation of the tacrolimus (Nayeri et al., 2017). Therefore, it is always best to discuss your usage of natural products with your pharmacist or doctor when you start (or stop) taking a supplement so that you can be monitored appropriately, as abruptly stopping a product that affects the metabolism of another drug could also affect your blood levels of that drug.

The effects of drugs with a narrow therapeutic spectrum can easily be altered by natural products. These are usually the drugs that doctors monitor in blood levels. Drug examples are digoxin, warfarin, valproic acid, phenytoin, tacrolimus, and thyroid medications. Other drugs that doctors do not monitor but that still have a narrow therapeutic spectrum are birth-control pills, some DOAC blood thinners, and antibiotics.

Fish oil and other medicinal oils seem to be very safe. Unlike traditional medications, they can be taken over a long period of time without adverse consequences. However, there have been reports of mercury contamination in fish oil pills (Foran et al., 2003). Mercury is described as a biochemical disruptor. A biochemical disruptor can hamper the production of energy and hormonal functions and cause nonspecific symptoms of bad health. Fish-oil manufactures are now on high alert to this concern, and improved products are now entering the market. Flaxseed oil is a vegetarian based omega-3 oil that does not have the same issue of mercury contamination.

CONCLUSION

Inflammation can cause havoc in our bodies. Anti-inflammatory drugs have side effects, especially when taken for long periods of time. But we are not powerless against inflammation. We can take control of our health and restore our bodies with natural products, lifestyle changes, and dietary changes. Although such changes are not easy, they are worth the effort.

6

STRENGTHENING THE IMMUNE SYSTEM

We are fighting an invisible war against pathogens. Pathogens are all around us, everywhere. Getting an infection can be like getting struck by lightning. Here are five things we can do to keep our immune system strong and avoid infection:

1. Reduce exposure to pathogens. Frequent hand washing, wearing a face mask, and social distancing are certainly ways to reduce exposure to pathogens, but don't forget that pathogens can be found in food, water, animal droppings, and in cooked or raw produce, meat, and plant products.

2. Sleep. Lack of sleep can increase susceptibility to the common cold (Cohen et al., 2009). Even more alarming, rats that were sleep-deprived died of sepsis (Rechtschaffen & Bergmann, 2002). People who travel and are at risk of not getting adequate sleep may benefit from taking melatonin. In addition, melatonin, the sleep hormone, might even have antiviral properties and benefits against viruses, including Covid-19 (Reiter et al., 2020; Silvestri & Rossi, 2013).

3. Nutrition. Adequate nutrition plays a vital role in keeping the immune system healthy. Four vitamin deficiencies are associated with frequently suffering from a colds or flu: vitamin A, vitamin D, vitamin E, and zinc. These vitamins play an integral role in keeping the immune system healthy (as discussed and cited below). Taking vitamin supplements yields miraculous benefits when a deficiency is restored to normal. Zoning in on people who are deficient in these four vitamins is the key to strengthening the immune system.

Let's recall risk factors for vitamin deficiencies:

- People who have conditions involving the gastro-intestinal tract: gastritis, GERD, swallowing issues, chronic nausea and vomiting, gastroparesis, gastric bypass, chronic diarrhea for any reason, colitis, and especially celiac disease.
- People who eat a limited diet: Those living in third-world countries, people who are institutionalized, picky eaters, vegans,

vegetarians, long-term ketogenic dieters, people with anorexia or an eating disorder.

- People with genetic defects, usually involving their biochemistry pathways. We cannot see these defects and are still discovering more about them. Sixty percent of people with sickle cell anemia also have a zinc deficiency. There are also phenotypes involving vitamin C and D.

- People with frequent exposure to toxins or chemicals. The U.S. Task Force (Institutes of Medicine (IOM) of the National Academies (formerly the National Academy of Sciences) stated that smokers have lower levels of vitamin C and should be taking a supplement. People who drink alcohol frequently often have multiple vitamin deficiencies, particularly B vitamins. People can have drug-induced vitamin deficiencies from prescription drugs.

4. Antivirals. In times of epidemics, vitamin C and zinc lozenges can double as antivirals when normal levels are elevated temporarily. This is a very rare occurrence and should only be used sparingly for short periods of time. Other natural products, including elderberry and Echinacea, also have antiviral activity, as well as lysine for cold and viral-related skin blisters. For statistical information on this issue, see (Siska, 2019).

5. Antibodies. Antibodies can be developed through using probiotics and taking vaccines. Antibodies are the magic bullets that kill pathogens. Vaccines give us the information to make the antibodies prior to the exposure. Certain probiotics can help vaccines work better, and the result is less susceptibility to a cold or flu, as well as fewer secondary opportunistic infections.

VITAMIN C

Marathon runners who took vitamin C had fewer colds (Gorton & Jarvis, 1999). Why single out marathoners? They are in constant motion and under physical stress, putting them at risk of dehydration and depleted electrolytes. Because vitamin C is water-soluble and involved in so many reactions throughout the body, perhaps it is quickly used up and washed out. Anyone at risk of low vitamin C levels from malnutrition, malabsorption, or physical stress might find it helpful to take extra vitamin C. Skiers and soldiers training in subarctic conditions also may

INVESTING IN YOUR HEALTH 71

benefit from vitamin C supplementation (Hemilä et al., 2013).

VITAMIN D

There are vitamin D receptors and activating enzymes on the surfaces of all white blood cells. The role that vitamin D plays in keeping the immune system healthy is complex because the immune system has to be perfectly balanced. If there is too much stimulation, autoimmune diseases can set in. If there is not enough immune system activity, frequent infections can result.

Low levels of vitamin D have been linked with both extremes, and low levels of vitamin D have been associated with worsening autoimmune diseases. Low levels of vitamin D are not the underlying cause of the autoimmune disease, but low levels of vitamin D can make autoimmune disease states worse (Szodoray et al., 2008).

Low levels of vitamin D have also been associated with frequent infections. The National Institutes of Health warned that low vitamin D levels are associated with frequent colds and influenza (NIH, 2009). It appears that vitamin D helps keep the immune system balanced, as does a gymnast walking on a balance beam. Since this 2009 NIH announcement, there have been many studies to determine the best regimen of vitamin D supplementation and to better understand this association (Martineau et al., 2017). Vitamin D daily or weekly is more effective than larger doses taken in a single dose or a once-a-month dose. The most common daily dose used was vitamin D3 300-4,000 IU (Camargo et al., 2020).

VITAMIN E

Vitamin E is most commonly known as a fat-soluble antioxidant. Vitamin E is similar to vitamin C in that it also plays a role in keeping the immune system healthy. Researchers are working hard to understand this role, but it appears that there are several mechanisms involved:

1. Reduction of PGE2 production by the inhibition of COX-2 activity mediated through decreasing nitrous oxide (NO) production.
2. Improvement of effective immune synapse formation in naive T cells and the initiation of T cell activation signals.
3. Modulation of Th1/Th2 balance. Higher natural killer cell activity and changes in dendritic function, such as lower IL-12 production and migration, were observed.

The best results were in male smokers who experienced a 69% lower incidence of pneumonia. This group smoked 5–19 cigarettes per day at baseline and exercised during leisure time. Also, elderly nursing home residents showed fewer upper respiratory infections and lower incidence of the common cold (Lee & Han, 2018).

More studies are needed to understand how vitamin E supplementation applies to school-aged children and healthy and well-nourished adults with optimal vitamin E levels. It is possible that these groups might not see a dramatic effect because a vitamin E deficiency would be less likely. Historically, it is usually people who have a vitamin deficiency that is then restored to normal who receive beneficial results from vitamin supplementation.

ZINC

Any person with a poor diet could have low levels of zinc and may benefit from a zinc supplement during the flu season. This includes people with anorexia, cachexia, or alcoholism, as well as strict vegetarians and those who have limited food choices for any reason (Bhutta et al., 1999). Also, most people with sickle sell anemia have a zinc deficiency due to genetics. Zinc deficiency affects 60% to 70% of adults with sickle cell disease (Prasad, 2002). Older adults in nursing homes also benefit from zinc supplementation, possibly due to poor appetite or diet, malabsorption, or a slowing of biochemical reactions (Meydani et al., 2007).

ANTIVIRALS

Timing is everything. The benefit has been greatest when started in the first 24 to 30 hours of onset of flu symptoms. Antivirals can reduce the severity of the flu and risk of complications and shorten the duration of the flu (Raus et al., 2015).

ZINC AS AN ANTIVIRAL

On rare occasions, a vitamin or a mineral can yield therapeutic effects when a normal level is elevated even higher. Zinc is one example. In the normal range, zinc keeps the immune system healthy, but at higher levels, it has antiviral properties against the flu and Covid-19 virus (Hemilä & Chalker, 2015; Velthuis et al., 2010).

There are various potentially appropriate dosages for zinc. The minimum dose for the average adult to avoid a deficiency is approximately 10 mg/day of elemental zinc. The maximum dose for the average adult—to avoid toxic effects such as nausea, vomiting, diarrhea, and immune dysfunctions—is 40 mg/day (NIH, ODS, 2020b).

The appropriate treatment dose for virally infected cells is 80–90 mg of zinc per day for short periods of time (one to three days). Long-term studies are needed to determine the ideal duration and dosage form (lozenges, capsules, or liquid). So far, we know that if levels go too high for too long, this can actually slow down and hamper the immune system, the opposite of the desired effect (NIH, ODS, 2020b).

High-dose IV zinc and vitamin C are being used experimentally in the fight against cancer (Dhawan & Chadha, 2010; Van Gorkom et al., 2019). Cancer cells are very similar to pathogens and virally infected cells. They are all cells that don't belong in our bodies, so our immune systems remove them. Zinc and vitamin C are major players when fortifying the immune system.

HIGH DOSES OF VITAMIN C AS AN ANTIVIRAL

Vitamin C at high doses (6–8 grams/day) has been shown to improve mortality in sepsis and to have positive clinical results in patients suffering from viral infections (Colunga et al., 2019; Marik, 2018). These high doses can cause side effects, such as kidney stones and diarrhea (Hemilä, 2017). Renal stones can result in renal damage, so they cannot be taken lightly. More studies are needed to see what else can happen when high doses are given for long periods of time. Because vitamin C is acidic, to protect the teeth from acidic damage, it should not be used as a lozenge or chewed in the gummy bear form.

ELDERBERRY

For short-term strengthening of the immune system, elderberry is an option. It increases the production of inflammatory cytokines, such as interleukins and the tumor necrosis factor. It should be used cautiously in situations where inflammation is already out of control because theoretically, elderberry could make the cytokine storm worse.

Elderberry, which has been compared with Tamiflu, is thought to have both antiviral and immunomodulating effects. Elderberry extract inhibits replication of several strains of influenza viruses A and B. In vitro, elderberry fruit extract also inhibits H1N1 swine flu. Elderberry flavonoids are thought to bind to H1N1 virions and to prevent the virus from entering host cells. Researchers also have found that people who have consumed elderberries have higher levels of antibodies against the influenza virus (Vlachojannis et al., 2010).

Commercial products are readily available, and people who have access to the fresh fruit can find online recipes for elderberry jams and syrups. The plant is generally safe for most people. Its medicinal properties are in the ripe fruit, but the seeds and other parts can cause nausea and vomiting.

ECHINACEA

Like elderberry, Echinacea possesses antiviral properties and immunomodulating effects. Certain products can increase the production of inflammatory cytokines, such as interleukins and tumor necrosis factor. Echinacea is similar to elderberry in that it can worsen a cytokine storm (Pleschka et al., 2009). A wide variety of Echinacea species, plant parts, preparations, and dosages are used, which leads to differing results; therefore, choosing an effective product is important (Karsch-Volk et al, 2015).

LYSINE

Lysine is an essential amino acid that releases growth hormone and also has antiviral properties. We have to get this amino acid from our diet because our body cannot manufacture it. Lysine is inexpensive, can be purchased without a prescription, and is available in generic form. To reduce recurrences of herpes simplex, the doses are 1000–3000 mg daily, which seems to reduce the severity and healing time.

Applying lysine topically also seems to help treat herpes simplex infection. For preventing canker sores, lysine 500 mg daily has been used. For treating canker sores, lysine 4000 mg daily in four divided doses has been used (Natural Medicines, n.d.).

OTHER ANTIVIRALS

Quercetin, a flavonoid found in onions, has antiviral properties. (Wu et al., 2015). Onions also have the unique ability to release gasses which make our eyes water when slicing them. These gasses have been studied for the purpose of disinfecting airborne pathogens. (Chang, et al., 2018). Covid-19 is in the air and wearing masks are a desperate attempt to control the spread of this virus. Some people use sliced onions throughout the home when a family member is sick. This unusual practice could potentially protect other family members from also getting sick.

Garlic, and oregano are also being studied for their antiviral and immune-fortifying properties.

DEVELOPING MORE ANTIBODIES WITH PROBIOTICS

As mentioned in the prior chapter, there is emerging evidence to suggest that probiotics can help a healthy immune system develop and mature. Specific probiotics given prior to vaccinations helped lead to higher antibody titers in response to the vaccination (Namba et al., 2010). The results of many randomized, controlled trials in classroom settings with school-aged children and young adults showed that those who received specific probiotics did not get the flu as frequently as did their classmates who were administered a placebo. Those who got probiotics and went on to develop the flu had shorter and less severe forms of the illness (Hao et al., 2015; King et al., 2014). Taking probiotic supplementation prior to receiving the influenza vaccination holds great promise for improving vaccine efficacy (Yeh et al., 2018). To choose specific probiotics products that have been shown to reduce flu, check a database that catalogs all the products on the market. AEProbio, Natural Medicines, and MedlinePlus show which products were tested for immune support and the level of evidence to support that product.

PROBIOTICS ARE NATURE'S ANTIBIOTICS

Probiotics are live organisms that compete one-on-one with pathogenic bacteria and fungi. It is important to chose the right probiotic for the right pathogen and to keep your expectations realistic. Probiotics usually work best for bacterial and fungal colonies in or around the gastro-intestinal (GI) tact. Probiotics are not effective against infections in peripheral locations: arm, legs, head, or feet. Life-threatening infections require medical treatment with proven antibiotics, antivirals, and antifungals when appropriate. This is one area where medicine, is truly the best medicine. Natural products are NOT a substitute for lifesaving medications.

Table 7. Pathogens and Probiotics

Pathogen(s)	Probiotic to oppose the pathogen	Reference
MRSA, Staph Aureus, Staphylococcus Aureus, Methacillin Resistant Staphylococcus Aureus,	Bacillus Subtillis, and possibly other Bacillus family members	(Piewngam et al., 2018)
C-diff, Clostridium Difficile	Many probiotics have been tested and used to prevent or treat CDI. The best studied probiotic agents in CDI are *Saccharomyces boulardii*, Lactobacillus GG (LGG) and other lactobacilli, and probiotic mixtures	(Katz, 2006; Surawicz, 2008)
H. Pylori,	The most used probiotic bacteria are Lactobacillus and Bifidobacterium	(Ruggiero, 2014)
Recurrent urogenital infections from yeast and bacteria with various names, including candidiasis	Most common is lactobacillus	(Abad & Safdar, 2009)

CONCLUSION

Fortifying the immune system with natural products is possible. Some people contract Covid-19, but they don't get any symptoms. This has also happened with the HIV and AIDS. Years later, they may test negative for the virus. It's as if their bodies had absorbed and annihilated the virus. How can we replicate this phenomenon? The answers are coming to us slowly.

7

THE MIND/BODY CONNECTION

There is a mind/body connection. Tapping into this is another piece to the health puzzle. Some people believe that mastering this area of health can control and repair all the other areas of health. A healthy mind is more than just having positive thoughts. Our mental health is the result of a three-way connection between our thoughts, our physical health, and our environment, which include our social environment. It's not only a connection between mind and body. It is actually a connection between mind, body, and environment connection.

MASTERING OUR THOUGHTS

Many scientists, including Dr. Bruce Lipton and Dr.

Candice Pert, are working to unravel the mysteries of how our thoughts affect our physical health. Their work suggests that our thoughts produce neurochemicals that are released into the bloodstream. These neuropeptides can become embedded into cell membranes and then control the DNA and ultimately the fate of the cell. In his book *Biology of Belief*, Dr. Bruce Lipton (2005) described this process in detail. Dr. Candice Pert's book is called *Molecules of Emotion: The Science Behind Mind-Body Medicine. (2010)*

I believe that self-loathing thoughts are the most dangerous to our health. If we could only replace those thoughts with love and compassionate for ourselves! I am living and learning and making mistakes just as is everyone else. It's OK to make mistakes because that is how we learn.

Forgiveness removes recurrent negative thoughts. After we forgive ourselves for not being perfect, we need to extend that forgiveness to others. We must understand that in this life, we have free will to help others or to harm them. It's our choice. We are not robots. This free will is how will live, learn, grow, and evolve. However, other people also have this free will, and sometimes they live, learn, and make mistakes at our expense. We must be OK with that possibility and forgive them because often they know not what they are doing. We must forgive to remove the recurrent negative thoughts that could sabotage our health.

Having a healthy environment to remove the source of negative thoughts. To have a harmonious environment, we must solve our social problems and strive to understand ourselves, as well as the people around us. To have a healthy mind-body-environment, we must be familiar with Maslow's hierarchy of needs and know how to get our needs met with integrity. To be authentic and genuine and to live with integrity is another secret to happiness. Many social problems seem to fade away when you do those two things and go with the flow. Also, realize that happiness is something to do, someone to love, and something to hope for. Happiness is also finding your place in the world where you are loved and appreciated for who you are.

Secret tip to finding exceptional health. Remove any perceived benefit to being sick. People have told me that they cannot get better because then their children will no longer come visit them, or they will lose some other sort of benefit. When they say that, I know that they are right; they cannot get better. My goal becomes making them as comfortable as possible so they can live with their disease until they are willing to forfeit that benefit and start the road to full recovery.

DON'T LET YOUR PHYSICAL HEALTH DERAIL YOUR MENTAL HEALTH

There are many ways our physical health can affect our mental health. Certain diseases such as diabetes, and lupus are closely linked to depression. These diseases can sabotage your mental health even if other parts of your mental health are perfectly in place. Gut health and systemic inflammation can also have an effect on our mood and behavior.

Probiotics for improved mood and mental health. We are now finding out that the gut and dysbiosis in the gut can worsen mental illnesses, including depression, psychosis, and schizophrenia. This is a quickly evolving area of medicine, and new discoveries are being made every day. Our gut is the manufacturing site of many neurotransmitters; 95% of serotonin is found in the gut (Cheung et al., 2019).

Probiotics can have an effect on our brain chemistry, mood, and behavior. Several probiotics are being marketed to alleviate anxiety and to promote a sense of calm. I would have to encourage anyone interested in this area to use a database that catalogs the probiotic products available on the market and the level of evidence for improved mental state or mood. As a reminder, the databases are AEProbio, Medline Plus, Consumer Labs, and Natural Database.

Turmeric has subtle anti-inflammatory properties and positive effects on the brain and mood (Ng et al., 2017). The exact mechanism is not completely understood, but can you imagine going through life with a brain on fire from inflammation? That has got to affect mood and behavior. More research is being done to understand curcumin's role.

Fish oils also have anti-inflammatory properties and double as a source of essential fatty acids. Fatty acids are necessary building blocks for brain matter and neurons. A relationship has been demonstrated between a balanced diet rich in omega-3 fatty acids, mood disorders, cognitive deterioration, and neurological diseases (Burhani & Rasenick, 2017).

Studies have shown that there is **increased blood flow** to the brain after high-dose omega-3 consumption (Jernerén et al., 2015). Is it possible that the omega-3s are redirecting the blood flow to needed areas much like eicosanoids and prostaglandins do for injuries? Omega-3s are similar in chemical structure to eicosanoids and other inflammatory mediators but without the inflammation. It is no wonder that fish oils are also being studied as cognitive enhancers.

A healthy mind is a balanced mind. For a healthy mind, all the neurochemicals must be in balance. For example, too much dopamine is associated with bad behavior, such as excessive gambling, compulsive shopping, sexual addictions, and impulsive decisions. These behaviors are common side effects from drugs that increase dopamine levels in the brain. Low levels of dopamine are also associated with restless leg syndrome, depression, and weight gain.

Too much serotonin is associated with a serotonergic reaction, including a fever, a frequent startle effect, anxiety, and insomnia. Low levels of serotonin are associated with lethargy, fatigue, apathy, anxiety, depression and insomnia.

It is best to give our body what it needs nutritionally to make the perfect amounts of neurochemicals and maintain a perfect balance. These neurochemicals are mainly made from amino acids and B vitamins (Briguglio et al., 2018; Glenn et al., 2019). These neurotransmitters control our mood, and to a certain extent our behavior. We should be getting our nutrients from food, but when that is not enough, vitamin supplements are an option.

L-Tryptophan is an amino acid that is converted to 5-HTP and that is then converted to serotonin and melatonin. Serotonin is the neurochemical that most anti-depressant drugs increase to produce positive effects. Sometimes depression sets in because our brain chemicals dry up. Anxiety, depression, and insomnia are closely related to serotonin levels. Consuming this amino acid directly translated to better mood (Lindseth et al., 2015). Consuming other amino acids (including tyrosine) that are needed to make other neurotransmitters (dopamine and catecholamines) have a more subtle effect on mood and behavior.

Vitamin B-complex. B vitamins are building blocks for many biochemicals in our brain and elsewhere in our bodies. Folic acid and vitamin B12 are involved in the synthesis of serotonin and other neurotransmitters. Vitamin B12 deficiency has been found in many patients with depression, decreased attention, decreased concentration, and decreased memory xxx (Kennedy, 2016; Olivera-Pueya & Pelegrin-Valero, 2017).

The same occurs with low folic acid levels. Folic acid deficiencies have also been associated with confusion, apathy, abulia, fatigue, and irritability (Kennedy, 2016; Olivera-Pueya & Pelegrin-Valero, 2017). In both folic acid deficiency and vitamin B12 deficiency, the intensity of the deficiency has been associated with the severity of the symptoms of depression and with the cognitive deficit associated with dementia (Kennedy, 2016). Observations are that many patients with folic acid deficiency may present a lower response to psychopharmacological treatment than those with normal levels. (Kennedy 2016; Olivera-Pueya & Pelegrin-Valero, 2017). Vitamin B6, also known as pyridoxine, has special importance as a precursor of serotonin and tryptophan, and can also play a role in mood and behavior (Olivera-Pueya & Pelegrin-Valero, 2017).

Magnesium is the relaxation mineral. It's used in a high dose IV form to relax the uterus and stop premature contractions in pregnant women. It's also used in high dose IV form following open heart surgery to relax the heart muscle and blood vessels. When taken orally in pill form, the effects are subtle and diarrhea is a drawback to getting high blood levels of it. Yes, milk of magnesia is a great laxative, but it is still the relaxation mineral that can also be added to hot bath water in the form of Epson salts (magnesium sulfate) to alleviate muscle tension.

Some people take their magnesium supplements at night because it can make some people sleepy.

The following is a chart of which neurotransmitters create which emotions and behaviors and the natural building blocks for that neurotransmitter. The last column is how we can intervene with natural products, mainly amino acids.

Table 8. Neurotransmitters

The neurotransmitter in our brain	The role it plays	The major building block for this neurotransmitter.
Serotonin (5-hydroxytryptamine, or 5-HT)	Optimism, happiness	L-tryptophan>serotonin>Melatonin
Gamma-aminobutyric acid (GABA)	calming neurotransmitter in the brain. GABA-a receptors for valium-like effect; GABA-b for muscle relaxer effect	Glycine, which resembles GABA in its action
Acetylcholine	autonomic nervous system, striatum, cortex, and hippocampus; M2 occurs in the autonomic nervous system, heart, intestinal smooth muscle, hindbrain, and cerebellum.	Choline and acetyl coenzyme
Dopamine	The feel good chemical. Associated with weight loss, and impulsive destructive behaviors: gambling, compulsive shopping, sexual addictions.	Tyrosine=found in aged cheese and red wine
Norepinephrine		Tyrosine is converted to dopamine, which is hydroxylated by dopamine beta-hydroxylase to norepinephrine.
Other Endorphins	Feel good chemicals	Vitamin B vitamins

COGNITIVE ENHANCERS

Any product that fortifies and strengthens the brain can potentially be a cognitive enhancer, including fish oils. (Abdullah et al., 2018; Sharma et al., 2015). Some of these products also provide benefits in other areas to strengthen overall health.

Ginseng is an ancient herb with many claims of longevity. Some people believe that it also has a positive effect on brain skills, including mood, behavior, and memory (Lee, Park, & Lim, 2011; Lee & Rhee, 2017). Panax ginseng (Asian ginseng) has an antioxidant property claimed to suppress Alzheimer's disease and similar pathologies. The intake of P. ginseng in healthy individuals is observed to increase the performance of memory performances (Suliman et al., 2016).

Rhodiola rosea is reported to improve cognitive function, enhance memory and learning, and protect the brain. (Suliman et al., 2016)

Ginkgo biloba is claimed to have neuroprotective effects observed in human and animals. A recent report has suggested the effect of Ginkgo biloba in treating Alzheimer's disease patient or other cognitive disorders. Ginkgo biloba also has been listed under group of antidementia drugs. It acts as antioxidant and antiapoptotic properties and also induces inhibition effects against caspase-3 activation and amyloid-β-aggregation toward Alzheimer's disease. (Suliman et al., 2016).

Arginine is another product with multiple longevity effects (Hu et al., 2017), and it also keeps the brain young (Gad, 2010). Arginine has the potential to preserve memory and the ability to learn. Arginine produces nitric oxide, which causes vaso-dilation of the micro-vascular. That means that it opens up the tiny blood vessels that supply blood and nutrients to the brain and other organs. Arginine is used in the IV form to preserve brain function in a medical condition called mitochondrial encephalopathy lactic acidosis (MELA), as well as in stroke-like episodes. MELA is a condition that causes young people to lose brain function. Arginine mitigates the loss of brain function and is often used in hospitals in an IV form to mitigate this horrible disease.

Arginine has been studied in treating other diseases of the brain with good results. It preserves the blood flow to the brain to improve brain function, but it cannot stop or reverse a disease process such as Alzheimer's (Anaeigoudari et al., 2015; El-Hattab et al., 2017; Paul & Ekambaram, 2011; Yi et al., 2009).

COMMONLY USED PRODUCTS

St John's wort is an herbal antidepressant with lots of drug interactions. But for someone young, healthy, and on no medications, it is an effective option. However, it can activate liver enzyme activity that can lead to the accelerated destruction of birth control pills and other sensitive drugs.

Cannabis is approved by the FDA to treat seizures in children. The information is coming rapidly about the medicinal proprieties of this herb. It appears that it is neuroprotective and may have more roles in medicine for Parkinson's disease, Huntington's disease, multiple sclerosis, and other conditions. (de Lago & Fernandez-Ruiz 2007).

There are many active ingredients in the original plant, and sorting out those individual chemicals and understanding their effects on the body will take time. People have been using this product for decades without serious side effects. It is commonly used for anxiety and stress management, and is much safer than alcohol for long-term use. If we could just switch the avid alcohol drinkers to cannabis, we could save a lot of money in health-care costs and avoid diseases such as cirrhosis and gastro-intestinal bleeds. But cannabis is not for everyone. Some people can have serious side effects from cannabis use. Side effects include psychosis, severe nausea, vomiting, and weight loss. All pharmacological drugs and herbal products are both good and bad. Cannabis is no exception.

There are many natural products on the market that may or may not help to improve brain function. I chose products that resonated with me and appeared in other parts of the book. I like products that restore several, not just one, area of health. I like knowing that the more I take these products for improved mood, and brain function, the healthier I am getting in all areas of my life. I also avoid products that could potentially throw brain chemistry out of balance or sabotage my health in other ways.

The following products I do not normally recommend because they don't seem to make the mind and body stronger and healthier over time, although they do seem to improve the mood in a temporary way while people work out their problems and find permanent solutions to the problems that are sabotaging their mental health. Under those circumstances, I do recommend the following products for temporary alleviation of symptoms. The following products can offer people hope and possibly prevent suicides.

Valerian root has been found to increase the amount of gamma aminobutyric acid (GABA) in the brain naturally, which can potentially help to calm anxiety. Benzodiazepine medications work this same way.

Kava kava root is an herbal product sold over-the-counter for its calming effect. Some side effects include headache, drowsiness, and diarrhea. Some forms of kava kava might cause liver damage. Because of this, kava kava has been banned in Germany, France, Switzerland, Australia, and Canada after 11 cases of kava kava-related liver injuries were reviewed. Four of these cases resulted in death.

Kratom (Mitragyna Speciosa) is a dangerous, but naturally occurring opioid agonist derived from the ground leaves of a tree that is native to Southeast Asia. It is killing people and is currently banned in several countries and US states, and is on the verge of being banned in many more. It is commonly used to mitigate the withdrawal symptoms associated with heroin and other opioids, but it seems to be addictive itself.

The reason why I take mental health so seriously and use various drugs and herbal products available on the market is because in 2015, in the United States, suicide was the seventh leading cause of death for males and the fourteenth leading cause of death for females (CDC, 2015). Additionally, suicide was the second leading cause of death for young people aged 15 to 34 and the third leading cause of death for those between the ages of 10 and 14 (NIMH, 2019).

Anyone considering suicide should reach out for profession help and cling to the belief that suicide is not the answer. It will not solve the problems or resolve the unlearned life lessons that could potentially follow people to an afterlife. It's best to solve these problems now with a professional's help and give yourself and others compassion and forgiveness.

CONCLUSION

People have been asking since the beginning of time why some people get sick while other people do not. I believe that there are many reasons. I believe that sometimes, it's a life lesson for us to learn how to take care of our bodies. For example, we must learn how to endure reality and not drink too much alcohol or indulge in too much junk food. Sometimes, it is just fate. It is our life lesson to understand and experience physical suffering and endure it. It is no fault of our own.

But fate is no reason to ignore the mind/body connection. Like all the other areas of health, a mind/body connection that is out of alignment can accelerate or worsen any situation or underlying disease. Finding great health must also involve having a healthy state of mind.

8

DETOXING THE BODY OF CHEMICAL DISRUPTORS

Detoxing is all about keeping our liver, kidneys, and intestines running in optimal condition so that our body can remove toxins quickly and effectively. The epic article "Hallmarks of Aging" refers to toxins as chemical disruptors that inactivate essential proteins, enzymes, and hormones. Toxins also can cause cell death, inflammation, oxidative damage, and premature aging (López-Otín et al., 2013).

The hung-over feeling that results from excessive alcohol consumption is an example of a buildup of toxins and the aftermath of exposure to toxins. It results in low energy, headache, and other unpleasant symptoms. But when the toxins leave the body and the body recovers naturally, energy levels go up, mood improves, and minor aches and pains go away.

Many people pursue regular detoxing and internal cleansing to maintain optimal health. It's natural to consume toxins from the environment occasionally. The problem occurs when we consume toxins faster than we can get rid of them or when our detoxifying organs malfunction. The obvious solution is to avoid the toxins in the first place. Prevention is key.

HEAVY METAL TOXICITY

Many mystery diseases are blamed on an accumulation of heavy metal toxins in the brain, nerves and other parts of the body. People living in highly polluted areas without regular access to clean air and clean water are at risk. People doing construction on old houses that contain lead paint are at risk. People who consume nonfood items, a condition called pica, are at risk. People who accidentally consume tainted food, tainted dietary supplements, or tainted drugs are at risk. Heavy metal poisoning presents itself as a mystery disease. Take for example these two cases that were reported in the *British Medical Journal* (Kew et al., 1993).

In the first case, the subject developed weakness and loss of sensation in his hands and feet after six weeks of starting a new herbal product. The symptoms progressed, so he went to the doctors, who noticed ridges in his fingernails and hyperkeratosis of the soles of his feet. The doctors also noted wasting of his limbs and no reflexes in his legs. After running several other tests, they checked his urine and found arsenic. They traced the source of the arsenic to the herbal supplement. The patient received treatment to remove the arsenic from his body, but unfortunately, he sustained permanent nerve damage and was still unable to work two years after the occurrence.

The second subject developed mystery symptoms after one week of taking the herbal product and finally went to his doctor four weeks after starting to take the supplement. This person was found to have mercury in his or her supplement instead of arsenic. This person developed GI symptoms, including loss of appetite, weight loss, and diarrhea. The symptoms progressed to changes in nerve sensations in the extremities and face, as well as tremors in his hands and sweating. The doctors discovered the person also had high blood pressure, rapid heart rate, anxiety, flushing, and reduced sensations in the fingers and toes from pinpricks. The case study did not mention treatment or the patient's recovery.

We can learn from these cases that poisoning from heavy metals can be insidious and gradual. It doesn't occur from a one-time accidental dose of something unless that dose happens to be an extremely high dose, in which case it is usually fatal. But low-dose poisonings can occur over weeks and present as mystery ailments.

Heavy-metal poisonings from dietary supplements can occur in products from other countries where there is less regulation over food and drugs and less government oversight of such things. Here in the USA, we have a government website called Medwatch that keeps track of such issues and warns the general public of tainted products and related problems.

Lead poisoning is a common occupational hazard for people working with lead pipes and lead paint. Blood lead levels from 25 and 60 μg/dL can produce neuropsychiatric effects, such as delayed reaction times, irritability, and difficulty in concentrating, as well as slowed motor nerve conduction and headaches. Anemia may appear at blood lead levels higher than 50 μg/dL. Abdominal colic involving paroxysms of pain may appear at blood lead levels higher than 80 μg/dL. High blood lead levels exceeding 100 μg/dL cause very severe manifestations, including signs of encephalopathy (a condition characterized by brain swelling), accompanied by increased pressure within the skull, delirium, coma, seizures, and headache (Wani et al., 2015).

Heavy metals have a strong attraction to brain and nerve tissues. Sometimes the accumulation of heavy metals can mimic psychiatric diseases. I recommend that anyone who is struggling with unexplained anxiety or other mental-health issues should have their heavy metals levels checked to rule out such toxicity as a possible cause of the symptoms.

INTERVENTIONS WITH NATURAL PRODUCTS

Severe symptoms of poisoning from heavy metals require medical treatment and supportive care. But a diet of whole foods, high-fiber foods, and foods that contain sulfur can keep the body free from an accumulation of toxins. Examples of whole foods that contain sulfur are broccoli, cauliflower, and asparagus. Here are some supplements that double as detoxifying agents.

Taurine and methionine are sulphur-containing amino acids. They are found in the cell membranes of excitable tissues in the brain and nerves. They decrease oxidative stress markers that result from exposure to heavy metals.

Alpha lipoic acid is a powerful antioxidant that regenerates other antioxidants (e.g., vitamins E and C, as well as reduced glutathione) and has metal-chelating activity. Both fat-soluble and water-soluble, it is readily absorbed from the gut and crosses cellular and blood-brain membrane barriers.

N-acetyl-cysteine (NAC) is an orally available precursor of cysteine. NAC is a chelator of toxic elements and may stimulate glutathione synthesis, particularly in the presence of vitamins C and E. This product also contains sulfur and has a pungent odor when in the liquid formulations used in hospitals.

Selenium is an important essential element that is present at a broad range of levels across populations. The selenide ion forms an extremely stable and insoluble compound with mercury and provides relief of mercurialism symptoms (Sears 2013).

THE DETOXING ORGANS AND HOW OUR BODIES REMOVE DANGEROUS CHEMICALS

- Excreted unchanged by the kidneys.
- Changed (metabolized) by the liver and then excreted by the kidneys.
- Excreted in the bile, into the intestines, and then eliminated through the gut.
- Excreted through the skin and hair.

- Emesis or diarrhea: We vomit them up or quickly expel them through the gut.
- Skin, nails, and hair—primarily for heavy metals.
- Lungs and exhalation of toxins.
- Future route: metabolization and breakdown by the probiotic gut bacteria and eliminated through the gut.

LIVER SUPPORT

Our liver is the primary site of many biochemical reactions. It is where excessive sugar is converted into fat before it is taken away to the periphery to be stored. It is also the location where toxins are inactivated before they can cause damage. People use the following supplements to support the liver and keep it running in prime condition: NAC, milk thistle, dandelion, turmeric, aspirin, and other supplements.

Many people say that they take one of these supplements prior to a heavy night of drinking and feel a noticeable difference the next day as far as having fewer hangover symptoms are concerned. However, most of the medical studies about such matters are conducted on people who already have liver damage, and at that point, these supplements don't have a noticeable empirical effect.

NAC is often used in hospitals to prevent liver

injury after a Tylenol overdose or exposure to some other toxin. It's also used sometimes to help cancer patients overcome the adverse effects that may be associated with toxic cancer drugs, such as isoffamide and cyclophosphamide. NAC is an immediate precursor to a very precious substance that our body makes called glutathione. Amino acids, such as cysteine, glutamate, and glycine, are also natural precursors from the food we eat.

Studies have measured glutathione levels going down after exposure to toxins. Damage occurs to the body and vital organs, usually involving the liver or kidneys, depending on the toxic exposure. Studies have also measured glutathione levels going up after NAC administration, with damage to vital organs mitigated.

Milk thistle, also known as silybin, is a high-profile product that is frequently in the medical news for its protective effects in preventing liver damage. However, just as with NAC, it is less likely to reverse the damage once it has occurred. Prevention is key.

Liver damage or liver failure is usually a slow process that occurs over long period of time and is closely connected to lifestyle and long-term consumption of toxins. The products discussed above do not restore or improve liver damage once it has occurred.

Some natural products can cause organ damage. Preventing exposure to toxins is key; if we want to stay healthy and have great energy, we should not be ingesting anything that can harm us. Illicit drugs and alcohol are obvious toxins, but some toxins are hidden in our supplements. However, sometimes even normally healthy supplements can trigger organ failure in people who are at risk. Sometimes a toxin is a vitamin or mineral that causes problems in elevated dosages or in combination with other toxins.

Niacin and vitamin A are common products that have been implicated in liver damage. Their potential adverse effects are widely known, yet often they are ignored. Technically, all pills are good and bad. Many natural products don't show up on lists of toxins, but they all have the potential to cause harm in high doses and under adverse circumstances.

Other less known herbal hepato-toxins are as follows. Chaparral leaf, laurie tridentate, creosote bush, grease wood, nordi-hydroguaiaretic acid (HDGA), jin bu huan, lycopodium serratum, levo-tetrahydropalmatine, germander, teucrium , hamaedrys, teucrium polium, kava, piper methysticum rhizome, mistletoe, viscum album, skullcap, scutellaria spp, symphytum (comfrey), senecio spp, crotalaria spp, heliotropium spp, maté (paraquay) tea, ackee fruit, atractylis gummifera, callilepsis laureola, cassia angustifolia, (senna), sassafras albidum, borago officinalis, pennyroyal , squawmint oil, hedeoma pulegoides, and mentha pulegium.

KIDNEY SUPPORT

The kidneys are responsible for removing toxins and other unwanted substances from our blood, including excess fluid that is no longer needed. However, we need water to dilute and carry the waste and toxins our of our body and make urine. When we are dehydrated, toxins become concentrated, and the blood pressure in our kidneys drops, so urine production slows. It's almost like a car engine without oil, and damage can occur. Our kidneys come to a halt. In some cases, irreversible kidney damage sets in.

Renal failure (kidney failure) can be like the perfect storm brewing. It's usually a combination of dehydration and poor blood flow through the kidneys due to sepsis or blood pressure medications or diuretics (AKA water pills). When a nephrotoxin is added to the situation, renal failure presents. The perfect storm has occurred. Kidney damage or kidney failure usually happens quickly and unexpectedly. Often it is reversible if caught early and treated with hydration and removal of offending agents. However, there are no known substances to reverse kidney damage once it has set in (Bouby et al., 2014).

NEPHROTOXINS

What is a nephrotoxin, you might ask? It's a trigger for renal failure. Here are some examples of normally healthy supplements that can cause renal failure in the setting of other contributing factors and in very high doses: vitamin D, chromium, creatine, vitamin C, and lysine. Vitamin D only causes renal failure when taken for long periods of time in excessive doses, such as 50,000 units daily or weekly, without blood monitoring. Under those conditions, it may cause too much calcium in the blood that deposits into the delicate renal tubules (Bouillon, 2020; Camargo et al., 2020). Vitamin C has caused kidney damage due to kidney stones that resulted from dosages of around 60 grams per day. That's 240 of the 250-mg pills (Gabardi et al., 2007). Renal damage from creatine, lysine, and chromium is more unpredictable, but usually it occurs like the perfect storm in conjunction with dehydration and low blood pressure in the kidneys.

GUT ILLUMINATION OF TOXINS

Many detoxing products on the market are laxatives. Flushing the toxins out of the intestines can feel refreshing, and that is one valid way to remove toxins and to detoxify. However, toxins can be reabsorbed and recycled into the bloodstream if they do not pass quickly out of the intestines. You may recall that my favorite laxative is magnesium pills, which double as an energy precursor and natural muscle relaxer.

PROBIOTICS FOR DETOXING

Many researchers have found out that the bacteria in the gut is like a mini-liver. It can break down toxins when liver and kidney failure have occurred. *E. coli* Nissle and others are being investigated to lower elevated ammonia levels in the blood. They change the toxic build-up of ammonia into something more beneficial. In the case of *E. coli* Nissle, it turns the ammonia into the amino acid arginine. The end result of taking these probiotics is lower ammonia levels in the bloodstream (Kurtz et al., 2019; Liu et al., 2018).

CONCLUSION

Many doctors will caution their patients not to take dietary supplements because so many things can go wrong. If you chose to take supplements, it's important to know what can go wrong so that you are on high alert and can intervene as soon as possible. It is also important to tell your doctor what you take so that he or she can conduct routine blood work that would detect any problem if it were to occur. It is best to use medicinal diets first to solve health issues and get our vitamins and minerals. When that is not enough, we can add natural products in pill and other forms. When that is not enough, we can add drugs. We should not be consuming products that don't have an indication. We should only consume products that serve a specific function.

9

OPTIMIZING BLOOD SUGARS, APPETITE CONTROL, AND WEIGHT LOSS

One of the best predictors of health and lifespan is a simple blood test called Hemoglobin A1c. The number from this test is the average blood sugar level over the past three months. With this number, researchers can predict the onset of the following diseases that normally occur with the passage of time. The longer and higher the A1c number is, the more likely it is that the following conditions will occur.

- Eye damage, such as cataracts and glaucoma, which may damage the blood vessels of the retina, potentially leading to blindness.
- Heart and blood vessel disease, stroke,

high blood pressure, and narrowing of the blood vessels (atherosclerosis). For men, erectile dysfunction may be a related issue.

- Nerve damage (neuropathy): tingling, numbness, burning, or pain that usually begins at the tips of the toes or fingers and gradually spreads upward. Eventually, you may lose all sense of feeling in the affected limbs.
- Damage to the nerves that control digestion, which can cause problems with nausea, vomiting, diarrhea, or constipation.
- Kidney damage, including irreversible end-stage kidney disease, which may require dialysis or a kidney transplant.
- Slow healing of cuts and blisters, which can become serious infections. Severe damage might require the amputation of a toe, a foot, or a leg.
- Hearing impairment.
- Skin conditions, including chronic and recurrent bacterial, viral, and fungal infections.
- Sleep apnea as a result of obesity, which may be the main contributing factor to both conditions. Treating sleep apnea may

INVESTING IN YOUR HEALTH

lower your blood pressure and make you feel more rested, but it's not clear whether it helps improve control of blood sugar.

- Alzheimer's disease, although its connection with blood sugar levels is not clear. The worse your blood sugar control, the greater the risk appears to be.
- Medical researchers and doctors can especially can see the damage to the tiny blood vessels in the back of the eye and how these changes correlate to blood sugar levels.

There is a linear pattern to high blood sugar and disease onset. The higher the blood sugar levels are and the more extended the length of time that the blood sugars are elevated, the sooner disease will occur. This pattern is most apparent by viewing the damage to the tiny blood vessels in the back of the eye. It is not easy to measure and view the onset of neurological damage or damage in other parts of the body, but damage in the back of the eye is easy to spot.

Some people don't take high blood sugar seriously because it feels good to have high blood sugar, and they don't want to make the lifestyle changes. It feels good to eat chocolate cake or drink surgery soda, but doing so is still damaging to our health. Having low blood sugar feels like crap, but that is what is healthiest for us. Naturally low blood sugar is good for us. Low blood sugar caused by drugs is a different story and can be dangerous because the body cannot compensate and bounce back. Hypoglycemia (an abnormal decrease in sugar in the blood) caused by drugs can be fatal.

The reason high blood sugar is so bad for us is that the sugar molecules (glucose) start to stick to healthy delicate tissues. It's like a watch that has syrup poured on it. It cannot function properly. The same thing happens in our bodies. The tiny blood vessels and nerve endings are the first to become permanently damaged. Then the damage starts to affect the larger blood vessels and nerves. In later stages, entire organs became dysfunctional, as in blindness, cardiovascular disease, dementia, kidney failure, and amputated feet from poor blood flow and chronic infections. Researchers describe this process as AGE molecules.

Another reason high blood sugar is so bad is insulin resistance. Insulin resistance occurs when the cell tries to reduce the constant influx of glucose (a term often used synonymously with blood sugar and technically the byproduct of sugar and carbohydrate metabolism). It is like a stove that burns wood being stuffed too full of wood. A stove that burns wood needs just the right amount of wood to burn hot. Too much or too little, and the internal system starts to malfunction. When the stove is stuffed too full of wood, the fire dies. There is not enough oxygen circulating through the stove, and the exhaust cannot be properly eliminated. Insulin resistance occurs when the door to the stove won't open to receive any more wood. On the surface of the cell membrane, the insulin receptors won't open to receive any more glucose. It's a protection mechanism.

Think of glucose as the wood. The insulin is the person carrying the wood and opening the door to the stove. The door on the stove is the insulin receptor. The stove is any kind of human cell. The solution is to consume less sugar and to exercise more. Exercise wakes up the cells and prompts them to burn the wood hotter and faster. Exercise and intermittent fasting are how you can get your cells to come alive.

RESET YOUR A1C WITH A SUITABLE FOOD ROUTINE

Getting healthy and slowing the aging process starts with taking control of our appetite and eating the right amounts of nutrient-dense foods. All the pillars of health fall into place as we can master this first step: eating suitable foods in suitable quantities.

The challenge is that if we don't plan our meals properly or if we get too hungry, our appetite causes us to be prone to making bad food choices. Also, many people are emotional eaters and have food addictions. These food addictions can be addressed through journaling or personal growth coaching. From a physical standpoint, part of the solution is to take control of our appetite with healthy proteins (amino acids), fiber, and healthy oils. Think of consuming these foods as preventative eating. Eating healthy proteins, fiber, and oils stabilizes our blood sugars and reduces food cravings.

Eating properly starts with willpower. However, there is usually a built-in time limit to willpower. It might last a week, a month, or even a year. In that time period, we must do our best to establish a proper routine so that when the willpower wears off, we are coasting on the automatic behaviors of our subconscious mind.

If we establish an automatic routine, then when we get hungry, we reach for the foods in our fridge and eat till we are satisfied. After a while, it doesn't matter to us whether we reach for an apple or an éclair. When we are in autopilot, we just do it. That's the beauty of the subconscious mind and automatic behavior. We need to tap into this built-in feature in our mind. We need to use it to our advantage.

Intermittent fasting. Think of intermittent fasting as fasting periodically throughout the day between meals and particularly between the last food of the day and the first food of the following day. Technically, this is not a fast, but it might feel like it. Imagine you had a protein smoothie for breakfast. A few hours later, you are hungry, but lunch is not for another three hours. Think of that time frame as an opportunity to fast. Some products to help you through the fast will be water, green tea, and ginger tea. Know that there is a lag time when our blood sugar drops, and then our liver starts to kick in and turn the adipose tissue into blood sugar that our body uses to make feel-good energy. Until that kicks in, we may be tempted to eat sugary foods for a quick fix. That lag time is different for all of us because it is actually the drop in insulin levels that liberates the fat from the adipose tissue. Sustained low blood sugar is what lowers insulin levels. Lower insulin levels trigger the release of adipose tissue (Rui, 2014).

Going through sugar and junk food detoxifying is like someone going through alcohol detoxifying. Over time, an active alcoholic becomes tolerant to the effects of alcohol, and then he or she must drink more to get the same ongoing effects from alcohol. The same thing happens with sugar. It's like a staircase that we walk up; at the top of the staircase is high blood sugars, high hemoglobin A1c, insulin resistance, and the diseases listed above. If we want to reverse the insulin resistance and lower our hemoglobin A1c, we must walk down the staircase, and that involves enduring a lower blood sugar level than we are accustomed to. After we get used to the lower blood sugar level, the negative sensations go away, and then we are able to repeat the process.

Fasting is only healthy for people with a healthy pancreas who are not on blood sugar medications. People with type 1 diabetes who are on blood sugar-lowering medications for type 2 diabetes must take a different approach and work with their doctor or dietitian because they are at risk of hypoglycemia. Hypoglycemia (an abnormal decrease in blood sugar) is very serious and can be dangerous. However, the good news for healthy people is that the more we practice intermittent fasting, the easier it becomes and the healthier we get.

To make fasting easier, I encourage people to drink more water. Drink water as if it were a prescribed natural product to help rest your Hemoglobin A1c. Green tea, ginger tea, and other herbal teas are also good options. Some people also use ginger essential oils to get through this lag time between meals. My favorite trick is to find something very engaging to do to distract my mind from the sensation of hunger. Examples would be going for a walk, chatting with a friend, or doing arts and crafts.

Preventative eating with protein powders and protein bars can help with between-meal food cravings. People often go to the pharmacy motivated to lose weight. They want to buy something to help them with this goal. Protein powders and protein bars are good options, but they are not necessary if one has a good diet and a good food routine. However, I find that using these protein bars and shakes simplifies life. It's great to have them in the car ready to go as emergency food to eat instead of fast food or junk food.

Proteins, fiber, and fats in the diet stabilize blood sugars and cause a sensation of satisfaction, often referred to as satiety. Choosing protein products varies a lot between individuals, based on taste preferences and food allergies. Yes, protein should taste good to you, but also it should not contain allergens that could sabotage your health. Many people are allergic to soy, wheat, dairy, or gluten. Fortunately, there are many products to choose from that accommodate various food allergies.

AMINO ACIDS

L-carnitine is an amino acid necessary for lipid metabolism and adipose storage and liberation. It is a compound similar to a vitamin that our bodies get from our diet. L-carnitine is the carrier of lipids into the mitochondria to go through betaoxidation and become ATP. Nothing else can do this except for l-carnitine. It is essential for life. Fortunately, other amino acids can convert into l-carnitine, so consuming meat or dietary supplements in pill form is not necessary.

L-carnitine is currently being studied for its positive effects in patients with type 2 diabetes (Bene, 2018).

GOOD OILS THAT CAN HELP: OLIVE OIL

Fats, also known as long-chain fatty acids, are the preferred form of energy for heart muscles and skeletal muscles because fats produce so much ATP (also known as adenosine triphosphate) or energy. One fat molecule produces more than 100 ATP, whereas one glucose or sugar molecule only produces a net of 2 or 3 ATP, depending on whether it is inside or outside the mitochondria. One bonus is that oils do not require insulin to get into the cells. Add bonus number two: oils and essential fatty acids double as the building blocks for cell membranes, skin, the brain, nerves, and other body organs.

Olive oil is the main culinary oil of the Mediterranean diet, which has amazing longevity effects and health benefits. To say that olive oil reduces Hemoglobin a1c would be a stretch, but replacing sugary foods with meats and vegetables cooked in olive oil: imagine the results (Romagnolo, 2017).

Oils and triglycerides are sometimes found in atherosclerosis deposits in the veins. Yes, they are found at the scene of the crime, but they are not the cause of it. Ask your doctor whether oils are healthy for you. Some people have certain diseases that can be exacerbated by oils. Oils are not for everyone, but for the average person, they seem to be beneficial, even essential for good health.

OTHER MEDICINAL OILS:

Fish Oils and Flax Seed Oil. Habitual use of fish oil seems to be associated with a lower risk of all causes of cardiovascular disease (CVD) mortality and also to provide a marginal benefit against adverse CVD events in the general population. The active ingredients in fish oils are the omega-3 oils. Flax seed oils are a vegetarian source of omega-3 oils. When these medicinal oils are part of a healthy food routine, added to salads and smoothies, they provide healthy calories, stabilize blood sugar, and increase longevity (Abbott et al., 2020; Li et al., 2020; Souza et al., 2020).

Wheat Germ Oil is high in vitamin E. Unlike synthetic vitamin E pills which only has one isolated form of vitamin E, wheat germ oil has all eight natural forms of vitamin E. This natural combination of vitamin E forms is one reason many experts say food sources of vitamins are safer than pill forms.

MCT OIL: WHAT NOT TO USE

A growing trend is to take MCT oil as a supplement. MCT oil is used in hospitals in the pediatric unit and the neonatal intensive care unit (NICU). MCT oil is very useful in children and babies who don't have any adipose tissue and are struggling to make energy. MCT enables these individuals to make ATP or energy more easily. MCT oil has the unique ability to enter the mitochondria without l-carnitine. It's also more readily absorbed from the gut into the bloodstream. Think of MCT oil as the oil version of sugar. It's converted into ATP quickly and easily.

However, I caution people who use MCT oil in large amounts to lose weight because it can bypass the need to convert the adipose tissue from around the belly area to energy. Keto dieters often use MCT oil because it might facilitate going into ketosis. It also might mitigate constipation. Despite the widespread use of MCT oil, the average dieter probably won't see the same benefit from it.

Similar to MCT oil are **Exogenous Ketone**

Supplements. They are also a source of energy and if used inappropriately can potentially mitigate weight loss or even cause weight gain. They are new on the market and we are still learning what the possible side effects and implications are from long term use and the side effects when used in diabetes and other disease conditions.

CONJUGATED LINOLEIC ACID (CLA)

Conjugated linoleic acid (CLA) is a dietary supplement found naturally in dairy products and beef that is sold as a weight-loss product. CLA appears to reduce body fat mass in animals, but results from human trials suggest that its effects are small. There are several red flags and reasons NOT to take CLA. It may help people lose weight, but it may not make them healthier. CLA also has been reported to increase insulin resistance and glycemia in obese men with metabolic syndrome. CLA has also been associated with pancreatitis and increased oxidative stress biomarkers (den Hartigh, 2019).

FIBER AND LOWER HEMOGLOBIN A1C:

Eating vegetables is the best way to get your fiber, but there are other viable options: fiber wafer crackers, fiber gummy bears, fiber drinks, fiber candy chews, and fiber pills of various contents. One common and affordable product is psyllium power, which can be mixed with water and consumed in beverage form. It is popular because it is less readily fermented, and it causes fewer abdominal problems. The way fiber works to lower glucose is by slowing access of glucose to the small intestine, delayed gastric emptying, and actions on carbohydrate digestion. Consumption of dietary fibers also lowers blood cholesterol levels and helps to normalize blood glucose and insulin levels (Marlett et al., 2002).

THE SEARCH FOR A MAGIC PILL

Researchers are looking for pills to mimic fasting and lower Hemoglobin A1c. They are experimenting with diabetic medications, particularly metformin in nondiabetic people to see whether it works to extend life. Many natural products can positively affect diabetes, including ginger, garlic, cinnamon, tarragon, bitter melon, fenugreek, and gurmar (Ota & Ulrih, 2017). However, there are two natural products in particular that I want to bring to everyone's attention: vitamin C and ginseng.

VITAMIN C

The chemical structures of vitamin C and glucose are very similar, and they compete for entry into the cell. Animals have the ability to convert glucose into vitamin C, but humans cannot do this. The effect that vitamin C has on diabetes and insulin resistance is very complex. Researchers are still trying to understand the relationship. Taking vitamin C at a dosage of 1000 mg/day or more yields a significant decrease in fasting blood sugar, triglyceride, LDL cholesterol, Hemoglobin A1c, and serum insulin: significantly good changes across the board. However, taking it at a dosage of 500 mg/day does not produce any changes (Afkhami-Ardekani & Shojaoddiny-Ardekani, 2007).

GINSENG

This product is an ancient herb that supposedly improves and extends life through various mechanisms. What does the medical literature say about Ginseng with regards to lowering Hemoglobin a1c? Several clinical trials and animal studies have demonstrated that ginseng and ginsenosides can lower blood glucose, increase insulin sensitivity, and regulate lipid metabolism. A meta-analysis of 16 randomized controlled trials in people with and without diabetes concluded that ginseng improved fasting blood glucose in people with and without diabetes significantly (Shishtar et al., 2014). Ginseng: Korean red ginseng (P. ginseng) and American ginseng (P. quinquefolius) have been used and studied. The part of the plant that is mainly used for medicinal purposes is the root. Additional potential health effects of ginsenosides include anticarcinogenic, immunomodulatory, anti-inflammatory, anti-allergic, anti-atherosclerotic, antihypertensive, and antidiabetic effects, as well as effects on the central nervous system (Christensen 2009).

CONCLUSION

Lower Hemoglobin A1c and weight loss go hand and hand. Many people use weight-loss products to lower their Hemoglobin A1c. Over-the-counter herbal products are not guaranteed to work because they are not tested by the Food and Drug Administration (FDA) for purity. Prescription diet pills are safer and more effective than over-the-counter products. The Obesity Society refers to them as an alternative to bariatric surgery. However, many people have side effects from these products, and they stop working after a while, after which the weight comes back.

In this chapter, I chose natural products that serve multiple purposes in bringing us back into alignment with our natural health. Weight loss, diabetes, and appetite control are hot topics.

10

ENERGY PRECURSORS ARE AN EMERGING AREA OF MEDICINE

Adenosine triphosphate (ATP) is the magic spark of life. ATP is a biochemical firecracker that is needed before an embryo's heart can start beating in its mother's womb. ATP is given to the embryo by its mother. Without it, life cannot exist at any stage. ATP is needed for muscle movement, organ functions, and repairs to damaged tissues. No wonder that longevity researchers have zoned in on the biochemistry of and the manufacturing process for this chemical. As we age, scientists can measure diminishing levels of ATP and other energy-related biochemicals in our bodies (Aunan et al., 2016; López-Otín et al., 2013).

In animal studies, particularly in studies of mice, researchers have observed that the decline of these energy precursors correlates with age-related disease.

They also have observed that restoring these precursors has the potential to reverse certain diseases. Researchers have been examining the energy precursor NAD+, which is an active form of niacin found at the end stages of ATP production. The high-profile research has been done by those such as Harvard professor David Sinclair, who discovered resveratrol, and this research is being funded by young Internet billionaires on a mission to reverse aging. They have discovered that NAD+ can play an integral role in reversing diseases, such as Alzheimer's, atherosclerosis, depression, diabetes, and retinal degeneration (Johnson & Imai, 2018; Martens et al., 2018).

But nowhere is the role of ATP and health more apparent than in the heart. The heart muscle is the organ that uses the most energy. It has the highest oxygen uptake rate and has the highest concentration of mitochondria in the body (Long et al., 2015). Some cardiologists are using energy building blocks to help patients with heart failure, and these cardiologists and their patients are seeing positive results and increased quality of life (Houston et al., 2018; Sinatra, 2015).

Ejection fraction (EF) is the scientific measurement used to measure the contraction and force of the heart muscle. EF is expressed as a percentage of how much blood the heart pumps out into the body with each contraction. In his book

Metabolic Cardiology, cardiologist Stephen Sinatra, MD, outlines case studies of patients who had life-changing results from starting natural supplements to promote ATP synthesis. With these products, he saw the EF increase from between 10% and 20% to between 40% and 50%. An EF fraction of 60% is normal, meaning that 60% of the total amount of blood in the left ventricle is pushed out with each heartbeat. An EF of between 10% and 20% means that the person has a mostly bedbound existence, with minimal movement. Sinatra also included case studies of people who stopped taking their energy precursor supplements, and their EF and quality of life went back to baseline, with an EF of 10% to 20%.

Energy precursor therapy (EPT) is being used in children with congenital mitochondrial dysfunction. Children with these congenital defects often have profound cardiac disease, cognitive/brain dysfunctions, and some of them had muscle pain and weakness. These are the organ systems that use the most energy. Doctors at the Kennedy Krieger Institute in Baltimore, Maryland, use EPT to improve and mitigate the condition but not cure the disease (Poling et al. 2016).

Certain types of migraines also respond to EPT (Shaik & Gan, 2015). Unlike the heart, the brain does not use mitochondria to make ATP. Instead, ATP is made in the surrounding fluid (the cytosol) through a less efficient, quicker, simpler method called hydrolysis. Therefore, the EPT for treating migraines is different from that of the heart (Shaik & Gan, 2015). Could energy precursors play a role in other types of disease states, such as chronic fatigue syndrome and fibromyalgia? Functional medicine physicians are experimenting with this possibility (Pizzorno, 2014).

WHAT DO THE EXPERTS SAY?

The Mitochondrial Medicine Society follows these trends. The experts in it are an international group of clinicians, physicians, and medical researchers working toward advancing education, global collaboration, and research in clinical mitochondrial medicine. They discuss how healthy and young mitochondria yield good energy and health. Mitochondria are factories or organelles that make ATP. Old mitochondria do not make ATP or energy efficiently. To boost old mitochondria and create new mitochondria, it is necessary to exercise and build muscle. Interval training, a technique of exercising fast, such as sprinting for 1 minute and then more slowly, like fast walking for 3 minutes, and repeating this for 30 minutes, twice a week, is a good example of how to activate new mitochondria (Parikh et al., 2009). The members of the Mitochondrial Medicine

Society have also discussed that providing the body with the building blocks for energy plays a vital role in creating new mitochondria and making adequate ATP. A healthy diet can also produce similar results. But when advanced age or disease is a factor, dietary supplements can help (see Tables 9 and 10).

It is important to note that energy-producing dietary supplements and EPT are not stimulants and do not act in the same way that caffeine would. Stimulants, such as caffeine or methamphetamines, push out the stored energy into the bloodstream and tissues. Stimulants provide short-term energy and then leave the body depleted of ATP. Coincidently, methamphetamine users have a very high rate of heart failure compared with members of the general public (Richards et al., 2018).

Table 9. Building Blocks and Supplements for Energy

Energy Precursors	Role of Function in Energy **Production**	Additional Information
CoQ10, ubiquinol for better absorption	Moves electrons around and is an antioxidant; found in every cell of the body, with high concentrations in the kidneys, liver, and pancreas	Q is a substance that our bodies make. Levels in a 70-year-old are about 50% of those in a 20-year-old.
B vitamins	Have many roles and are building blocks for other energy biochemicals and antioxidants, such as Niacin, which is intimately involved in ATP synthesis	Commonly put in energy shots; NAD+ is an active form touted as a cure for aging. These vitamins have upper limits set by the FDA that should not be exceeded.
Creatine	Makes ATP and carries it to where it is needed	Found in high amounts in the brain and muscles; commonly used by bodybuilders
L-carnitine	Semi-synthetic amino acid found in red meat; lysine and other amino acids can be converted into L-carnitine, which carries fat particles into the ATP factory (mitochondria) and removes excess, potentially toxic acyl compounds and lactic acid.	Also used by fertility doctors to increase libido and sperm motility
Alpha lipoic acid	A substance our bodies make that has antioxidant properties with an affinity for fat molecules in membranes and nerves	Concerns exist about rare adverse thyroid effects in high doses.
Vitamin C	Moves electrons around to make ATP and also protects membranes from damage as antioxidant	Plays other longevity roles in the body, such as collagen formation in the skin and immune system support
Vitamin E	Thought to control oxidative damage to the mitochondrial membrane	Antioxidants are used to preserve the mitochondrial membranes that facilitate electron transfers. Rogue, flay-away electrons damage the mitochondrial membrane.
Phosphate	Three of these molecules make up each ATP molecule.	Too much is dangerous and can cause deposits into soft tissues. A healthy body easily gets what we need from food. Supplementation is only needed in cases of alcoholism, malnutrition, and other disease states. A simple blood test will tell whether supplementation is needed.
Magnesium	Found in energy drinks; it is involved in many biochemical processes in our bodies.	Truly a powerful substance that makes every situation better though various mechanisms
D-ribose	The sugar that begins the metabolic process for the production of ATP	Effective for improving the heart's tolerance to ischemia in patients with coronary artery disease.

ADP indicates Adenosine triphosphate.

Table 10. Traits of Energy Cocktails of Natural Supplement Regimens
Use by functional medicine doctors for energy, general good health, and vitality in people 50 years and older or those with declining health: acetyl-l-carnitine (500 to 1,000 mg, twice a day); alpha-lipoic acid (100 to 200 mg, twice a day); B-complex vitamins (daily), Coenzyme Q10 (100 to 200 mg a day); D-ribose (5 g, once or twice a day); magnesium (150 to 300 mg, twice a day); and NADH (5 to 10 mg a day) (Pizzorno, 2014)
Use for congenital mitochondrial dysfunctions: highly variable and patient-specific, depending on the type of defect; tests are performed to determine the type of congenital defect, and then a product regimen is prescribed. (Poling et al. 2016)
Use for headaches: magnesium oxide (400 mg, twice a day) and riboflavin (200 mg, twice a day) (Shaik & Gan, 2015)
Use in heart failure: CoQ10 (90 to 150 mg a day); d-ribose (5 gm a day); magnesium 400 mg a day; and l-carnitine (500 to 1000 mg a day) (Houston et al., 2018; Sinatra 2015)

DRAWBACKS OF ENERGY PRECURSORS

All pills can cause harm. It is important to know what can go wrong with these products, to be on high alert for these occurrences, and if they do occur to take quick corrective action. Sinatra (2015) speculated in his book that certain types of arrhythmias are caused by and accelerated when ATP levels in the heart get too high or low. Energy levels should be in the natural zone and restored in balance with the other energy precursors. Energy drinks and shots of high-dose B vitamins have been associated with fatal cardiac conditions (Mangi et al., 2016).

Also consider mitochondrial apoptosis and mitochondrial hormesis. Hormesis means that the intervention or supplement is a double-edged sword. It has bad and good effects. Poljsak (2016) discussed in an epic article hallmarks of aging through mitochondrial apoptosis and hormesis. Apoptosis occurs when the mitochondria self-destruct when the cell becomes defective. Restoring energy precursors could potentially bypass this innate system. There is a concern that some of these products can lead to cancer if these energy precursors get too high or low (Poljsak 2016).

There is also a possibility that the prostate-specific antigen, which is a marker of prostate cancer, could rise after starting nicotinamide adenine dinucleotide therapy for longevity purposes. Therefore, it is too early and experimental to recommend energy precursors for otherwise healthy people. Those who have symptoms of an ATP deficits, such as heart failure, migraines, or low energy levels should only take these supplements under the watchful eye of a physician.

11

HORMONES AND LONGEVITY

There are basically two types of hormones in our bodies: hormones that build our bodies and hormones that tear our bodies down. Hormones that build our bodies are released mostly during states of relaxation and sleep. Examples are growth hormone, thyroid hormone, parathyroid hormone, insulin, and all the sex hormones, including testosterone, progesterone, estrogen, and DHEA. Hormones that tear our bodies down are the stress hormones, such as corticosteroids (also known as prednisone), adrenalin, and epinephrine. High levels of these hormones are associated with bone breakdown and muscle breakdown because they put us in a survival state in which routine maintenance of the body is deferred to focus on surviving. The breakdown of our stored resources is necessary to get us out of the crisis, but under chronic stress, the crisis remains ongoing, and our body therefore ages prematurely. This is why many experts recommend that we get our stress under control if we want to live longer and in optimal health.

Regarding longevity (living longer), experts at the Endocrinology Society have said: Keep the levels in the normal range. Natural is best. If it is not broken, don't intervene. Hormones are like vitamins. They need to be in the natural zone; levels that are too high or too low can cause problems.

Table 11. Symptoms of Hormones that are Too Low or Too High		
Hormone	Too Low: Symptoms	Too High: Symptoms
Thyroid	Fatigue, sensitivity to cold, constipation, dry skin, weight gain	Rapid heart rate, insomnia, irritability, sensitivity to heat
Testosterone	Fatigue, obesity, loss of body hair, loss of libido, loss of muscle mass	Oily skin, increased red blood cell count, blood clots, accelerated cardiovascular disease, more facial and body hair.
Estrogen	Depression, migraines, mood swings, hot flashes, painful sex, increase in urinary tract infections (UTIs)	Bloating, swelling, blood clots
Progesterone	Depression, migraines, low libido	Weight gain, insulin resistance, blood clots
Growth hormone	Injuries that won't heal	Excessive bone growth, accelerated cardiovascular disease, enlargement of abdominal organs
Parathyroid hormone	Tingling in the lips, hands, fingers, and toes. Twitching, muscle cramps, and pain	Fragile bones, kidney stones, excessive urination, bone and joint pain
Adrenal hormones	Fatigue, sleep disturbances	Mood changes, bloating, weight gain, insulin resistance
Vitamin D	Brittle bones, low calcium levels, high parathyroid levels, low energy, chronic and nonspecific pain without injuries, more frequent colds and flu. Accelerated autoimmune diseases	High calcium and phosphate levels in the blood. Calcium and phosphate deposits in the soft tissues, including kidneys, and kidney damage

Hormones have a feedback mechanism. They turn on and off when needed, based on signals from other parts of the body. Also, hormones resist going out of the normal range. If they go out of the range for too long, bad things will happen. Take for example testosterone. If levels go too high, the body will change it into another less harmful hormone, such as estrogen, to reduce testosterone levels. High levels of testosterone are associated with accelerated cardiovascular disease.

Something similar happens with the thyroid. If a normal person takes thyroid supplements to elevate normal thyroid levels even higher (in an attempt to lose weight), the body will make less thyroid hormone to keep the levels in the healthy and normal range. Experts say that it is OK to increase a low hormone level to the high end of the normal range for improved health and greater longevity. But if you want to live longer and live disease-free, experts say not to go above the high end of the normal range.

Female hormones are more complicated. There is no normal range for estrogen or progesterone. Take for example the fluctuations that occur during a menstrual cycle or the fluctuations during pregnancy. All those levels are normal. Therefore, there is no standard level for doctors to aim for. Most doctors replace female hormones based on how the patient feels and once their symptoms improve or resolve.

According the Endocrinology Society, replacing the sex hormones, including testosterone, is optional. It's not required to live longer. So many doctors will give patients the choice. And I believe that choice is best made by the patient and the doctor together, after taking into considerations the potential risks and benefits.

Many women choose not to use estrogen products for fear of cancer. They go through menopause naturally and endure any symptoms. Some women use natural products to alleviate symptoms of menopause, but the concern for cancer is always there. There are no guarantees, not even with natural supplements. Some women chose to replace estrogen and progesterone to keep their bones strong and to preserve their cognitive function. They are at low risk for cancers and blood clots, and they are willing to take the risks associated with hormone replacement. Experts have said that women who benefit the most from hormone replacement are those younger than 60 years of age within 10 years of the onset of menopause who show no treatment contraindications. Women older than 60 years of age have more risk factors and more complications (NAMS, 2017).

Another thing to consider when deciding whether to take female hormones is that too much progesterone is associated with weigh gain. It's like the testosterone that causes men to bulk up with muscles, except progesterone causes women to bulk up with adipose. Estrogen is associated with increased risk of blood clots and cancers. Women who supplement with testosterone can also get acne and facial hair in the jaw area.

Growth Hormone. Perhaps we should rename this hormone the growth and REPAIR hormone. This hormone helps us grow to our adult size, but once we are adults, it helps to repair injuries and the normal wear and tear that occur during daily activities. It is released at night when we sleep as part of our natural rhythm. Its release is also stimulated by the intake of amino acids that are found in mother's milk. As we age, we produce increasingly less growth and repair hormone. The body wears down faster than it can repair itself, which is when old age starts to set in. The cartilage in our knees does not regenerate quickly enough, and the joints become bone on bone. Our spinal column loses strength, and we develop spinal stenosis and other age-related conditions. The list goes on and on, including osteoporosis.

But just as with all other hormones, more is not necessarily better. We need just enough growth hormone to grow to our adult size and then just enough to maintain the repairs to our body because of something called hormesis. Hormesis is a double-edged sword.

GROWTH HORMONE, ANABOLIC HORMONES, AND HORMESIS: THE DOUBLE-EDGED SWORD

Anabolic hormones, such as growth hormone and testosterone, are popular because they have been linked to benefits such as increased muscle mass, decreased fat accumulation, preservation of brain function, thicker skin, and improved healing from wounds and injuries. But these hormones are like a double-edged sword: They yield quality of life at the cost of quantity of life. Scientists call this phenomena hormesis (Calabrese et al., 2014).

Growth hormone and the amino acids that release growth hormone are fascinating because they are also repair hormones and amino acids. Growth hormone gives our body the equivalent of a shoeshine every night to keep our bodies in good condition. But too much is associated with shorter lives. Also, less growth hormone is associated with a longer life (Junnila et al., 2013). The life span of mice, worms, and flies was extended by 50% when their growth hormone was in the low end of the normal range (Junnila et al., 2013). Incidentally, people with the longevity gene to live past 100 years old are often short in stature. Very tall people or those with high levels of growth hormone usually die prematurely. Think of Andre the Giant, who died at age 46 of heart failure. This information has led some people to reduce their growth hormone levels through calorie restriction. Scientists say that these people are extending their lives, but their quality of life is going down because they are also experiencing muscle atrophy, diminished sex drive, and brain atrophy. Another downside to growth or anabolic hormones is that things can grow, including cancers, such as breast cancer (Murphy et al., 2020). In medical literature, the growth and repair hormone is also referred to as insulin-like growth factor. Those two terms are often used interchangeably by scientists.

Table 12. Commonly Used Hormonally Active Products (Ask a medical doctor for advice.)		
Type of Hormone	Name of Dietary Supplement	Comments
Thyroid	Iodine, keto stuff, dried-up animal thyroid glands (various manufacturers)	Restoring thyroid levels to normal can result in fuller and thicker hair.
Adrenal fatigue	Rest. Reduce stress. Meditate.	A real condition that we test for in hospitals with cosyntropin. We treat with prednisone and dexamethasion.
Male sex	Androstenediol, Androstenedione, Chrysin, DHEA (Dehydroepiandrosterone), Oats (Avena sativa), Tribulus (Tribulus terrestris)	The body resets high levels of testosterone and changes it to estrogens.
Bone health	Vitamins D2, D3, D4 essential for life; essential for bone health	The parathyroid hormone forces the calcium into the bone, but available only by Rx
Female sex	Alfalfa (Medicago sativa), bio-identical hormones, Black cohosh (Actaea racemosa), Chasteberry (Vitex agnus-castus), DHEA (Dehydroepiandrosterone), Dong quai (Angelica sinensis), Flaxseed (Linum usitatissimum), Hops (Humulus lupulus), Kudzu (Pueraria lobata), Licorice (Glycyrrhiza glabra), Panax ginseng, Red clover (Trifolium pratense), Sage (Salvia officinalis), Soy (Glycine max), Wild yam (Dioscorea villosa), Phytoestrogens [aka plant estrogens], isoflavones, lignans, and coumestans	phytoestrogens bind to estrogen receptors to alleviate menopausal symptoms but do not have estrogen effects.
Insulin (High levels cause difficulty losing weight. We want the levels naturally low and the receptors sensitive.)		Insulin levels must drop (as a result of sustained low blood sugar) before the body converts fat into energy.
Growth and repair	Arginine, lysine, (other amino acids that convert to arginine and lysine: ornatine, citrulline)	Low levels of growth hormone are associated with longevity. High levels are associated with better and more youthful physical state.
Libido enhancers	Arginine, ginseng, l-carnitine, acetyl l-carnitine. Also fenugreek, yohimbi, Stronvivo, dehydroepiandrosterone (DHEA), maca, and Zestra	For a boost in libido
Pregnancy HCG	HCG oral and sublingual solutions available.	For weight loss. The body quickly makes antibodies to neutralize it, and it stops working. Not recommended as a long-term solution for weight loss. Works by liberating fat independent of insulin levels

Osteoporosis is an inevitable condition associated with the passage of time. Bones are constantly breaking down and building up. Over time, the breakdown is more accelerated than the build-up, and osteoporosis sets in. Hormones that keep the bones decrease in volume. Hormones that keep the bones strong are estrogen, testosterone, growth hormone, and the parathyroid hormone. The parathyroid hormone's job is to take the calcium in the bloodstream and deposit it into the bones, making the bones stronger. All the calcium pills in the world are going to do NOTHING for your bones unless the hormones are in place to deposit the calcium in the bones. This is why I do not recommend taking a calcium supplement to keep bones strong (Siska, 2017). An exception is that a deficiency in vitamin D or a calcium deficiency will accelerate osteoporosis, so under those conditions, I do recommend calcium and vitamin D supplements. Testosterone, growth hormone, DHEA, and estrogen can stop bone loss and potentially build bone up (Cannarella et al., 2019). However, prescription drugs are very effective at treating osteoporosis without increasing hormonal risks.

CAN ANYTHING TURN BACK TIME?

The following list of natural products contains my best recommendations to preserve bone mass, lower blood sugar, preserve cognitive function, preserve muscle mass, and decrease body fat. The side effect from taking these products is increased libido, like what was present during youth. You may recognize many of these products from other chapters because they work on restoring other areas of health as well, and some of them are technically not hormonally active products. But the potential net effect is a younger state of being. Without using drugs, these are my best recommendations for healthy people to slow the passage of time.

Arginine helps preserve several areas of health, such as enhancing blood sugar, cognitive functions, muscle and fat composition, and injury recovery (Gad, 2010). Arginine is an amino acid found in milk that stimulates the release of the growth and repair hormone (Chromiak & Antonio, 2002). Other amino acids, such as citrulline, can change in to arginine if needed. Arginine can change into ornithine if levels become too high. Sometimes ornithine is added to amino acid combinations to enhance the effectiveness of the arginine, but there is controversy as to whether ornithine releases growth hormone on its own. Arginine has the added effect of increasing microvascular blood flow. It dilates the tiny blood vessels in our skin and other organs though nitrogen oxide activity. Many people believe that this is why it has such a powerful effect on increasing libido and treating erectile dysfunction.

Lysine also releases growth hormone and is

an amino acid that is often used in combination with arginine. Arginine can accelerate a viral outbreak of skin lesions, such as herpes, fever blisters around the mouth, and shingles. Lysine mitigates this side effect by competing with arginine for entry into the cells. Lysine also has antiviral properties. In addition to that, lysine is the only other amino acid that causes the release of growth hormone that we know of for sure without a doubt.

Ginseng is an ancient herb (Shin et al., 2020). American ginseng and Panas ginseng contain ginsenosides and polysaccharides. These affect hormones (estrogen levels) and blood glucose levels, among other effects (Natural Medicines, 2020). Ginseng has long been used as a cognitive enhancer, as noted in previous chapters. Ginseng has been reported to have aphrodisiac properties. Data from animal studies have shown a positive correlation between ginseng, libido, and copulatory performances, and these effects have been confirmed in case-control studies in humans (Leung & Wong, 2013). You may recall that ginseng can increase dopamine levels. Dopamine is thought to be connected with desire. Acetylcholine is involved in arousal, and the neurotransmitter GABA is connected with orgasm. Ginseng has been shown to increase extracellular dopamine and acetylcholine in rat brains (Shi et al., 2013). `L-carnitine` is an amino acid that is essential for energy production and lipid metabolism. It also has effects on the reproductive system. Many fertility doctors use it with great success. When compared with testosterone, carnitines provided significantly more activity in improving erectile functions without affecting the size of the prostate (Cavallini et al., 2004). The male participants who took testosterone suffered the adverse effect of enlargement of the prostate, in addition to which, there were concerns about cardiovascular disease (Morden et al., 2019). Many men do not take testosterone supplements due to the concerns of prostate enlargement and cancer, but there are other more natural options.

Any one of these supplements alone could improve libido, but what about taking all three of them together? Someone had already thought of that and went a step further and added two types of l-carnitine forms. They used arginine, ginseng, l-carninine, and acetyl-carnininte (Morgante et al.,

2010). (Lysine is optional to control viral outbreaks.) Carnitines exist in many different forms in the body. Acetyl-carnitine is thought to have better central nervous system activity than l-carnitine, which is most active peripherally. Researchers found a significant improvement in sexual satisfaction in the group that used all four supplements compared with the placebo group (Morgante et al., 2010). Increased libido indicates that these products are indeed turning back the hands of time.

12

UNDERSTANDING HOW THESE TEN AREAS AFFECT OUR HEALTH

W hen one of the 10 areas discussed in the preceding chapters come out of alignment, it can either cause a disease, accelerate an already existing disease, or it can have no effect at all. A pattern that you may have noticed is balance: the balance of hormones, neurochemicals, vitamin levels, energy precursors, and others biochemicals. I also recommend balance in our personal lives. The balance of exercise and rest. The balance of self-care and care of others. The balance of work and play. The balance of exercising the mind and exercising the body. The balance of consuming healthy foods and consuming UNhealthy comfort foods. Many people say at the end of their lives that what they will miss most is eating ice cream or some other sort of "happy food." For that reason, I never discourage the consumption of "happy food" in moderation. Experiencing joy is one reason why we are alive.

Therefore, we must work at a gentle pace to achieve a sustainable healthy and balanced lifestyle. If the changes are too extreme and severe, that abrupt or forced change can sabotage our efforts. The goal should be to incorporate healthy changes into our lifestyle gently that translate to automatic and effortless habits. It starts with knowledge of how our health works and understanding how much of an impact that these changes can make.

It is my belief that people are NOT lazy; they just don't believe that the changes will make an impact in their lives. They are not convinced that the work is worth it relative to the outcomes for them. But health is wealth. Without good health, other areas of our lives disintegrate: our careers, our relationships, and our finances. People with healthy lifestyles and sound food routines are often resistant to disease and infection. They have great mood and energy. They sleep well, they eat whole foods, and they play sports and enjoy fun physical activities. They are most free of pain, and they may show off their amazing health with flattering clothing. They take natural supplements to slow the aging process and to maintain excellent health and energy. We are all living, learning, loving, and evolving.

Improving our health starts with loving ourselves

INVESTING IN YOUR HEALTH

just the way we are in the present moment. It also involves forgiving ourselves for not having taken better care of our health in the past. It takes understanding that we are all doing the best we can under the circumstances that we are in. You are probably reading this book because you desire better health and want to slow the aging process. Thank you for finding me, and thank you for sticking with me this far. I wish you the best of luck and success with your health journey. There is much medical information out there. The question you should be asking yourself is: Which information applies to me? Which information will result in better health in my situation? Which of the 10 areas of health is my weakest link due to genetics or lifestyle? Most of the information on the internet on how to optimize health is true; it's just not true for everyone. Finding out which information is true for you is your job. It involves tuning into your intuition and using your discernment.

For example, some people say that eggs and the cholesterol in them are bad. Cholesterol accelerates atherosclerosis and is found in clogged blood vessels. But I say that although cholesterol is found at the scene of the crime, it is not to blame. Cholesterol is only bad for certain people with a disease process, possibly systemic inflammation affecting the lining of the blood vessels. Cholesterol is trying to protect the blood vessel linings from further damage and sudden occlusion (blockage). Therefore, the statement that eggs and cholesterol are bad for you should really be restated: Eggs are only bad for certain people. Doctors know who these people are and will tell you if you ask which foods are best for your medical condition. If they don't give you any dietary restrictions, the Mediterranean diet is thought to have the most longevity effects for the average person.

FUTURE BOOKS THAT I AM NOW WORKING ON

I am working on a future book about medicinal diets, recipes with super foods, grocery lists, and cooking hacks for people with families, growing kids, picky eaters, and mature adults. Stay tuned for that. Also stay tuned for another book called *Journaling for Better Health*. It is designed to help you discover the mental blocks that are sabotaging your ideal food routine and healthy lifestyle. Yes, you do have all the answers inside you! You can overcome and conquer your food addictions and unhealthy habits.

The fourth medical book that I am writing is called *Hospital Confidential*. It explains what you need to know before you go into the hospital. How to read your medical chart, what questions to ask your doctor and nurses to make sure you get the best

WHAT I TRIED TO ACCOMPLISH FOR YOU IN THIS BOOK

I have presented the information the best I could. I did not mention every single product or medical intervention ever used or talked about because I had to use my intuition and discernment to set priorities for the information that I had. I chose products that I though had the biggest impact and applied to most people regarding the products that are readily available on the market and affordable. This book is my opinion of how I see that we can optimize health based on peer reviewed medical data. I honor the opinions of others and I realize that there are more than one path to great health.

The 10 areas talked about in this book are the areas in which we can intervene with natural products. Doctors who have access to medications are able to intervene in additional areas, such as declogging arteries that become occluded with plaque over time. Similar to an old house with bad plumbing pipes, our arteries develop atherosclerosis with the passage of time. Although a whole-foods diet, certain herbs, teas, and other lifestyle interventions can help, prescription drugs also can accomplish this goal. We have statins, and now we have seek-and-destroy drugs called monoclonal antibodies to do this effectively and completely. As a hospital pharmacist, I believe in using the best medicine available for a disease process.

I hope you found this information helpful and enlightening. I hope it encourages you to live a better, healthier, happier, more successful life that resonates in other areas. I truly wish you well. Life is precious. Enjoy it while you can. Go out there and live while you are alive. I wish everyone around the world a healthy, happy life with the people they love.

I would like to thank and acknowledge Theodore Roosevelt for his brilliant and insightful quotation, which gave me the courage to publish this book:

It is not the critic who counts; not the man who points out how the strong man stumbles, or where the doer of deeds could have done them better. The credit belongs to the man who is actually in the arena, whose face is marred by dust and sweat and blood; who strives valiantly; who errs, who comes short again and again, because there is no effort without error and shortcoming; but who does actually strive to do the deeds; who knows great enthusiasms, the great devotions; who spends himself in a

INVESTING IN YOUR HEALTH

worthy cause; who at the best knows in the end the triumph of high achievement, and who at the worst, if he fails, at least fails while daring greatly, so that his place shall never be with those cold and timid souls who neither know victory nor defeat.

— THEODORE ROOSEVELT (1909)

REFERENCES

- Abad, C. L., & Safdar, N. (2009). The role of lactobacillus probiotics in the treatment or prevention of urogenital infections: A systematic review. *Journal of Chemotherapy*, *21*(3): 243–252. doi:10.1179/joc.2009.21.3.243
- Abbott, K. A., Burrows, T. L., Acharya, S., & Thota, R. N., Garg M. L. (2020, June 13). DHA-enriched fish oil reduces insulin resistance in overweight and obese adults. *Prostaglandins, Leukotrienes, and Essential Fatty Acids*, *159*: 102154. doi:10.1016/j.plefa.2020.102154
- Abdullah, M., Jowett, B., Whittaker, P. J., & Patterson, L. (2019, March). The effectiveness of omega-3 supplementation

in reducing ADHD associated symptoms in children as measured by the Conners' rating scales: A systematic review of randomized controlled trials. *Journal of Psychiatric Research, 110*: 64–73. doi:10.1016/j.jpsychires.2018.12.002

- Afkhami-Ardekani, M., & Shojaoddiny-Ardekani, A. (2007). Effect of vitamin C on blood glucose, serum lipids, & serum insulin in type 2 diabetes patients. *Indian Journal of Medical Research, 126*(5): 471–474.

- Agustin, M., Yamamoto, M., Cabrera, F., & Eusebio, R. (2018, June 7). Diffuse alveolar hemorrhage induced by vaping. *Case Reports in Pulmonology*: 9724530. doi:10.1155/2018/9724530

- American Diabetes Association. (2019). Anti-inflammatory drug, used for decades, now found to lower blood glucose levels in people with type-2 diabetes. (Press Release).

- American Heart Association. (2020). *Home page*. Retrieved from www.heart.org

- Ametov, A. S., Barinov, A., Dyck, P. J., Kozlova, N., Litchy, W. J., Low, P. A., . . . Ziegler, Z. (2003). The sensory symptoms of diabetic polyneuropathy are improved with alpha-lipoic acid: The Sydney Trial. *Diabetes Care, 26*: 770.

- Anaeigoudari, A., Shafei, M. N., Soukhtanloo, M., Sadeghnia, H. R., Reisi, P., Nosratabadi, R., . . . Hossein, M. (2015, September 28). The effects of L-arginine on spatial memory and synaptic plasticity impairments induced by lipopolysaccharide. *Advanced Biomedical Research, 4*: 202. doi:10.4103/2277-9175.166138

- Aunan, J. R., Watson, M. M., Hagland, H. R., & Søreide, K. (2016). Molecular and biological hallmarks of ageing. *British Journal of Surgery, 103*: e29–e46. doi:10.1002/bjs.10053

- Ayala, F. R., Bauman, C., Cogliati, S., Leñini, C., Bartolini, M., & Grau, R. (2017, March 16). Microbial flora, probiotics, *Bacillus subtilis*, and the search for a long and healthy human longevity. *Microbial Cell, 4*(4):133–136. doi:10.15698/mic2017.04.569

- Black, R. E. (2003). Children in third world countries and zinc: Zinc deficiency, infectious disease, and mortality in the developing world. *Journal of Nutrition, 133*: 1485S–1489S.

- Balbi, M. E., Tonin, F. S., Mendes, A. M., Borba, H. H., Wiens A., Fernandez-Llimos F., & Pontarolo R. (2018, March 14). Antioxidant effects of vitamins in type 2 diabetes: A meta-analysis of randomized controlled trials. *Diabetology & Metabolic Syndrome, 10*: 18. Retrieved from www.ncbi.nlm.nih.gov/pubmed/29568330

- Bene, J., Hadzsiev, K., & Melegh, B. (2018, March 7). Role of carnitine and its derivatives in the development and management of type 2 diabetes. *Nutrition & Diabetes, 8*(1): 8. doi:10.1038/s41387-018-0017-1

- Bhutta, Z. A., Black, R. E., Brown, K. H., Meeks-Gardner, J., Gore, S., Hidayat, A., . . . Shankar, A. (1999, December 1). Prevention of diarrhea and pneumonia by zinc supplementation. *Journal of Pediatrics, 135*(6): 689–697. doi:10.1016/S0022-3476(99)70086-7

- Blot, W. J., Li, J. Y., Taylor P. R., Guo W., Dawsey S, Wang, G. Q. . . . Li, G. Y. (1993). Malnourished men in China and Multivitamins: Nutrition intervention trials in Linxian, China: Supplementation with specific vitamin/mineral combinations, cancer incidence, and disease-specific mortality in the general population. *Journal of the National Cancer Institute, 85*: 1483–1492. Retrieved from PubMed.

- Bouby, N., Clark, W. F., Roussel, R., Taveau, C., & Wang, C. J. (2014). Hydration and kidney health. *Obesity Facts, 7*(Suppl 2):19–32. doi:10.1159/000360889

- Bouillon, R. (2020). *Vitamin D and extraskeletal health.* UpToDate (online). Retrieved from: http://www.uptodate.com/contents/vitamin-d-and-extraskeletal-health

- Boyle, R. J., Robins-Browne, R. M., & Tang, M. L. K. (2006, June 1). Probiotic use in clinical practice: What are the risks? *The American Journal of Clinical Nutrition, 83*(6), 1256–1264. Retrieved from academic.oup.com/ajcn/article/83/6/1256/4632996

- Braakhuis, A. J., & Hopkins, W. G. (2015). Impact of dietary antioxidants on sport performance: A review. *Sports Medicine, 45*: 939. Retrieved from https://doi.org/10.1007/s40279-015-0323-x

- Briguglio, M., Dell'Osso, B., Panzica, G,

et al. (2018, May 10). Dietary neurotransmitters: A narrative review on current knowledge. *Nutrients*, *10*(5): 591. doi:10.3390/nu10050591

- Burhani, M. D., & Rasenick, M. M. (2017). Fish oil and depression: The skinny on fats. *Journal of Integrated Neuroscience*, *16*(s1): S115–S124. doi:10.3233/JIN-170072

- Calabrese, V., Scapagnini, G., Davinelli, S., Koverech, G., Koverech, A., De Pasquale, C., Trovato Salinaro, A., . . . Genazzani, A. R. (2014). Sex hormonal regulation and hormesis in aging and longevity: Role of vitagenes. *Journal of Cell Communication and Signaling*, 8(4): 369–384. doi:10.1007/s12079-014-0253-7

- Camargo, C. A., Sluyter, J., Stewart, A. W., Khaw, K.-T., Lawes, C. M. M., Toop, L., Waayer, D., & Scragg, R. (2020, July 15). Effect of monthly high-dose vitamin D supplementation on acute respiratory infections in older adults: A randomized controlled trial. *Clinical Infectious Diseases*, *71*(2): 311–317. doi:10.1093/cid/ciz801

- Cannarella, R., Barbagallo, F., Condorelli, R. A., Aversa, A., La Vignera, S., &

REFERENCES

Calogero, A. E. (2019, October 1). Osteoporosis from an endocrine perspective: The role of hormonal changes in the elderly. *Journal of Clinical Medicine, 8*(10): 1564. doi:10.3390/jcm8101564

- Cavallini, G., Caracciolo, S., Vitali, G., Modenini, F., & Biagiotti, G. (2004, April). Carnitine versus androgen administration in the treatment of sexual dysfunction, depressed mood, and fatigue associated with male aging. *Urology, 63*(4): 641–646. Retrieved from https://www.ncbi.nlm.nih.gov/pubmed/15072869

- Centers for Disease Control (CDC). (2015). *Suicide facts at a glance.* Retrieved from www.cdc.gov/violenceprevention/pdf/suicide-datasheet-a.pdf

- Chang, Yeoung Seuk Bae, Il Sheob Shin, Hyun Jin Choi, Ji Hyun Lee, Ji Weon Choi. Microbial Decontamination of Onion by Corona Discharge Air Plasma during Cold Storage. *Journal of Food Quality: Nonthermal Plasma for Food Quality and Safety* [online] https://www.hindawi.com/journals/jfq/2018/3481806/

#introduction Published November 18, 2018. Accessed August 10, 2020.

- Cheung, S. G., Goldenthal, A. R., Uhlemann, A. C., Mann, J. J., Miller, J. M., & Sublette, M. E. (2019, February 11). Systematic review of gut microbiota and major depression. *Front Psychiatry*, *10*: 34. doi:10.3389/fpsyt.2019.00034

- Christensen, L. P. (2009). Ginsenosides' chemistry, biosynthesis, analysis, and potential health effects. *Advances in Food and Nutrition Research*, 55: 1–99. doi:10.1016/S1043-4526(08)00401-4

- Cizginer, S., Ordulu, Z., & Kadayifci, A. (2014). Approach to Helicobacter Pylori infection in geriatric population. *World Journal of Gastrointestinal Pharmacological Theory,* *5*(3): 139–147. doi:10.4292/wjgpt.v5.i3.139

- Cohen, S., Doyle, W. J., Alper, C. M., Janicki-Deverts, D., & Turner, R. B. (2009). Sleep habits and susceptibility to the common cold. *Archives of Internal Medicine*, *169*(1): 62–67. doi:10.1001/archinternmed.2008.505

- Colunga-Biancatelli, R. M. L., Berrill, M., & Marik, P. E. (2020, February). The antiviral properties of vitamin C. *Expert*

Review of Anti-Infective Therapy, 18(2): 99–101. doi:10.1080/14787210.2020.1706483

- Chromiak, J. A., & Antonio, J. (2002). Use of amino acids as growth hormone-releasing agents by athletes. *Nutrition,* 18(7–8): 657–661. doi:10.1016/s0899-9007(02)00807-9

- Daily, J. W., Yang, M., Park, S. (2016). Efficacy of turmeric extracts and curcumin for alleviating the symptoms of joint arthritis: A systematic review and meta-analysis of randomized clinical trials. *Journal of Medicinal Food, 19*(8): 717–729. doi:10.1089/jmf.2016.3705

- de Lago, E., & Fernandez-Ruiz, J. (2007). Cannabinoids and neuroprotection in motor-related disorders. *CNS & Neurological Disorders, 6*(6): Epub. doi:10.2174/187152707783399210

- den Hartigh, L. J. (2019, February 11). Conjugated linoleic acid effects on cancer, obesity, and atherosclerosis: A review of pre-clinical and human trials with current perspectives. *Nutrients, 11*(2): 370. doi:10.3390/nu11020370

- Dhawan, D. K., & Chadha, V. D. (2010). Zinc: A promising agent in dietary chemoprevention of cancer. *Indian Journal of Medical Research, 132*(6): 676–682.

- El-Hattab, A. W., Almannai, M., & Scaglia, F. (2017). Arginine and citrulline for the treatment of MELAS syndrome. *Journal of Inborn Errors in Metabolic Screening*, 5: Epub. doi:10.1177/2326409817697399
- Foran, S. E., Flood, J. G., & Lewandrowski, K. B. (2003, December). Measurement of mercury levels in concentrated over-the-counter fish oil preparations. *Archives of Pathology and Laboratory Medicine, 127*(12): 1603–1605.
- Frijhoff, J., Winyard, P. G., Zarkovic, N., Davies, S. S., Stocker, R., Cheng, D., . . . Ghezz, P. (2015). Clinical relevance of biomarkers of oxidative stress. *Antioxidant Redox Signal, 23*(14): 1144–1170.
- Gabardi, S., Munz, K., & Ulbricht, C. (2007). A review of dietary supplement-induced renal dysfunction. *Clinical Journal of the American Society of Nephrology, 2*: 757–765.
- Gad, M. Z. (2010, July). Anti-aging effects

of l-arginine. *Journal of Advanced Research*, *1*(3): 169–177.

- Glenn, J. M., Madero, E. N., & Bott, N. T. (2019, June 12). Dietary protein and amino acid intake: Links to the maintenance of cognitive health. *Nutrients*, *11*(6): 1315. doi:10.3390/nu11061315
- Gorton, H. C., & Jarvis, K. (1999). The effectiveness of vitamin C in preventing and relieving the symptoms of virus-induced respiratory infections. *Journal of Manipulative and Physiological Therapeutics*, *22*(8): 530–533.
- Hao, Q., Dong, B. R., & Wu, T. (2015, February 3). Probiotics for preventing acute upper respiratory tract infections. *Cochrane Database of Systematic Reviews*, *2015*(2): CD006895.
- He, H. Y., Liu, M. Z., Zhang, Y. L., & Zhang, W. (2017). Vitamin harmacogenomics: New insight into individual differences in diseases and drug responses. *Genomics Proteomics Bioinformatics*, *15*(2): 94–100. doi:10.1016/j.gpb.2016.10.005
- Hemilä, H. (2017, March 29). Vitamin C

and infections. *Nutrients*, *9*(4): 339. doi:10.3390/nu9040339

- Hemilä, H., & Chalker, E. (2015, February 25). The effectiveness of high-dose zinc acetate lozenges on various common cold symptoms: A meta-analysis. *Biomedical Central Family Practice*, *16*: 24. doi:10.1186/s12875-015-0237-6

- Hemilä, H., Chalker, E., Johnston, C. S., Barkyoumb, G. M., & Schumacher, S. S. (2013). Vitamin C and the common cold: Vitamin C for preventing and treating the common cold. *Cochrane Database of Sytematic Reviews*, *2013*(1): CD000980.

- Hill, M. J. (1997). Intestinal flora and endogenous vitamin synthesis. *European Journal of Cancer Prevention, 6*: S43–S45.

- Houston, M., Minich, D., Sinatra, S. T., Kahn, J. K., & Guarneri, M. (2018). Recent science and clinical application of nutrition to coronary heart disease. *Journal of the American College of Nutrition*, *37*(3): 169–187. doi: 10.1080/07315724.2017.1381053

- Hu, S., Han, M., Rezaei, A., Li, D., Wu, G., & Ma, X. (2017). L-arginine modulates glucose and lipid metabolism in obesity and diabetes. *Current Protein & Peptide Science*, *18*(6), 599–608. doi:10.2174/1389203717666160627074017

- Institute of Medicine, Food and Nutrition Board. (2000). *Dietary reference intakes for vitamin C, vitamin E, selenium, and carotenoidsexternal link disclaimer.* Washington, DC: National Academy Press, 2000.
- Institute of Medicine, National Academies. (n.d.). *Dietary Reference Intakes (DRIs).* Retrieved from:

http://www.nationalacademies.org/hmd/~/media/Files/Activity%20Files/Nutrition/DRI-Tables/6_%20Elements%20Summary.pdf?la=en and http://www.nationalacademies.org/hmd/~/media/Files/Activity%20-Files/Nutrition/DRI-Tables/7_%20Nutrients%20Summary.pdf?la=en

- Jernerén, F., Elshorbagy, A. K., Oulhaj, A., et al. (2015, July). Brain atrophy in cognitively impaired elderly: The importance of long-chain ω-3 fatty acids and B vitamin status in a randomized controlled trial. *American Journal of*

Clinical Nutrition, 102(1): 215-221. doi:10.3945/ajcn.114.103283

- Johnson, S., & Imai, S. I. (2018). NAD + biosynthesis, aging, and disease. *F1000 Research, 7*: 132. doi:10.12688/f1000research.12120.1

- Junnila, R. K., List, E. O., Berryman, D. E., Murrey, J. W., & Kopchick, J. J. (2013). The GH/IGF-1 axis in ageing and longevity. *Natinal Review of Endocrinology, 9*(6): 366–376. doi:10.1038/nrendo.2013.67

- Karsch-Völk, M., Barrett, B., & Linde, K. (2015, February 10). Echinacea for preventing and treating the common cold. *Journal of the American Medical Association, 313*(6): 618–619. doi:10.1001/jama.2015.17145

- Katz, J. A. (2006). Probiotics for the prevention of antibiotic-associated diarrhea and *Clostridium difficile* diarrhea. *Journal of Clinical Gastroenterology, 40*: 249–255.

- Kennedy, D. O. (2016, January 27). B vitamins and the brain: Mechanisms, dose, and efficacy: A review. *Nutrients, 8*(2): 68. doi:10.3390/nu8020068

- Kew, J., Morris, C., Aihie, A., Fysh, R.,

Jones, S., & Brooks, D. (1993). Arsenic and mercury intoxication due to Indian ethnic remedies. *British Medical Journal*, 306(6876): 506–507.

- Khaerunnisa, S., Kurniawan, H., Awaluddin, R., Suhartati, S., & Soetjipto, S. (2020). Potential inhibitor of Covid-19 main protease (M^{pro}) from several medicinal plant compounds by molecular docking study. *Preprints*, 2020030226. doi:10.20944/preprints202003.0226.v1

- Khansari, N., Shakiba, Y., & Mahmoudi, M. (2009). Chronic inflammation and oxidative stress as a major cause of age-related diseases and cancer. *Recent Patents on Inflammation and Allergy Drug Discovery, 3*(1): 73–80. doi:10.2174/187221309787158371

- King, S., Glanville, J., Sanders, M. E., Fitzgerald, A., & Varley, D. (2014). Effectiveness of probiotics on the duration of illness in healthy children and adults who develop common acute respiratory infectious conditions: A systematic review and meta-analysis. *British Journal of Nutrition, 112*(1): 41–54. doi:10.1017/S0007114514000075

- Kleszczynski K., & Fischer, T. W. (2012).

Melatonin and human skin aging. *Dermatoendocrinology, 4*(3): 245–252. doi:10.4161/derm.22344

- Kurtz, C., Millet, Y., Puurunen, M., et al. (2019, January 16). An engineered *E. coli* Nissle improves hyperammonemia and survival in mice and shows dose-dependent exposure in healthy humans. *Science Translational Medicine, 11*(475): Epub. doi:10.1126/scitranslmed.aau7975

- Lee, G. Y., & Han, S. N. (2018, November 1). The role of vitamin E in immunity. *Nutrients, 10*(11): 1614. doi:10.3390/nu10111614

- Lee, S. H., Park, W. S., & Lim, M. H. (2011). Clinical effects of Korean red ginseng on attention deficit hyperactivity disorder in children: An observational study. *Journal of Ginseng Research, 35*(2): 226–234. doi:10.5142/jgr.2011.35.2.226

- Lee, S., & Rhee, D. K. (2017). Effects of ginseng on stress-related depression, anxiety, and the hypothalamic-pituitary-adrenal axis. *Journal of Ginseng Research, 41*(4): 589–594. doi:10.1016/j.jgr.2017.01.010

- Leung, K. W., Wong, A. S. (2013). Ginseng and male reproductive function.

Spermatogenesis, 3(3): e26391. doi:10.4161/spmg.26391

- Li, Z. H., Zhong, W. F., Liu, S., Kraus, V. B., Zhang, Y. J., Gao, X., Lv, Y. B., . . . Mao, C. (2020, March 4). Associations of habitual fish oil supplementation with cardiovascular outcomes and all causes of mortality: Evidence from a large population-based cohort study. *British Medical Journal, 2020*: 368. doi:10.1136/bmj.m456

- Lindseth, G., Helland, B., & Caspers J. (2015). The effects of dietary tryptophan on affective disorders. *Archives of Psychiatric Nursing, 29*(2): 102–107. doi:10.1016/j.apnu.2014.11.008

- Lipton, B. (2005). *The Biology of belief: Unleashing the power of consciousness, matter, and miracles.* Carlsbad,CA: Hay House.

- Liu, J., Lkhagva, E., Chung, H. J., Kim, H. J., & Hong, S. T. (2018). The pharmabiotic approach to treat hyperammonemia. *Nutrients, 10*(2): 140. doi:10.3390/nu10020140

- Long, Q., Yang, K., & Yang, Q. (2015). Regulation of mitochondrial ATP synthase in cardiac pathophysiology. *American*

Journal of Cardiovascular Disease, 5(1): 19–32.

- López-Burillo, S. L., Tan, D. X., Mayo, J. C., Sainz, R. M., Manchester, L.C., & Reiter, R. J. (2003). Melatonin, xanthurenic acid, resveratrol, EGCG, vitamin C, and alpha-lipoic acid differentially reduce oxidative DNA damage induced by Fenton reagents: A study of their individual and synergistic actions. *Journal of Pineal Research, 34*(4): 269–277.

- López-Otín, C., Blasco, M. A., Partridge, L., Serrano, M., & Kroemer, G. (2013). The hallmarks of aging. *Cell, 153*(6): 1194–1217. doi:10.1016/j.cell.2013.05.039

- Lundberg, G. D. (2015, May 11). Magnesium deficiency: The real emperor of all maladies? Medscape. Retrieved from: http://www.medscape.com/viewarticle/844214

- Mangi, M. A., Rehman, H., Rafique, M., & Illovsky, M. (2017). Energy drinks and the risk of cardiovascular disease: A review of current literature. *Cureus, 9*(6): e1322. doi:10.7759/cureus.1322

- Marik, P. E. (2018, November 14). Hydrocortisone, ascorbic acid, and thiamine (HAT) therapy) for the treatment of sepsis: Focus on ascorbic acid. *Nutrients, 10*(11): 1762. doi:10.3390/nu10111762

- Marlett, J. A., McBurney, M. I., & Slavin, J. L. (2002). Position of the American Dietetic Association: Health implications of dietary fiber. *Journal of the American Dietetic Assocociation, 102*(7): 993–1000. doi:10.3390/nu11020370

- Martens, C. R., Denman, B. A., Mazzo, M. R., Armstrong, M. L., Reisdorph, N., McQueen, M. B., . . . Seals, D. R. (2018, March 29). Chronic nicotinamide riboside supplementation is well-tolerated and elevates NAD+ in healthy middle-aged and older adults. *Nature Commununications, 9*(1): 1286. doi:10.1038/s41467-018-03421-7

- Martineau, A. R., Jolliffe, D. A., Hooper R. L., et al. (2017, February 15). Vitamin D supplementation to prevent acute respiratory tract infections: systematic review and meta-analysis of individual participant data. *British Medical Journal, 356*: i6583. doi:10.1136/bmj.16583

- Mayo, J. C., Tan, D. X., Sainz, R. M., Natarajan, M., López-Burillo, S., & Reiter,

R. J. (2003). Protection against oxidative protein damage induced by metal-catalyzed reaction or alkylperoxyl radicals: Comparative effects of melatonin and other antioxidants. *Biochimica et Biophysica Acta (BBA): General Subjects, 1620*(1–3): 139–150.

- McBride, J. (2000, August 2). B12 deficiency may be more widespread than thought. Retrieved from: https://www.ars.usda.gov/news-events/news/research-news/2000/b12-deficiency-may-be-more-widespread-than-thought/
- Meydani, S. N., Barnett, J. B., Dallal, G. E., Fine, B. C., Jacques, P. F., Leka, L. S., & Hamer, D. H. (2007, October). Serum zinc and pneumonia in nursing-home elderly. *American Journal of Clinical Nutrition, 86*(4):1167–1173. doi:10.1093/ajcn/86.4.1167
- Montilla-López, P. L., Muñoz-Agueda, M. C., Feijóo López, M., Muñoz-Castañeda, J. R., Bujalance-Arenas, I., Túnez-Fiñana, I. (2002). Comparison of melatonin versus vitamin C on oxidative stress and antioxidant enzyme activity in Alzheimer's disease induced by okadaic

acid in neuroblastoma cells. *European Journal of Pharmacology, 451*(3): 237–43.

- Morden, N. E., Woloshin, S., Brooks, C. G., & Schwartz, L. M. (2019, March 1). Trends in testosterone prescribing for age-related hypogonadism in men with and without heart disease. *Journal of the American Medical Association Internal Medicine, 179*(3): 446–448. doi:10.1001/jamainternmed.2018.6505
- Morgante, G., Scolaro, V., Tosti, C., Di, Sabatino A., Piomboni, P., and De, Leo, V. (2010). Treatment with carnitine, acetyl carnitine, l-arginine and ginseng improves sperm motility and sexual health in men with asthenopermia. *Minerva Urology and Nefrology, 62*(3): 213–218. Retrieved from www.ncbi.nlm.nih.gov/pubmed/20940690
- Mounce, B. C., Cesaro, T., Carrau, L., Vallet, T., & Vignuzzi, M. (2017). Curcumin inhibits Zika and chikungunya virus infection by inhibiting cell binding. *Antiviral Research, 142*: 148–157. doi:10.1016/j.antiviral.2017.03.014
- Muntwyler, J., Hennekens, C. H., Manson, J. E., et al. (2002). Well-nourished males: Vitamin supplement use in a low-risk population of U.S. male physicians and

subsequent cardiovascular mortality. *Archives of Internal Medicine, 162*: 1472–1476.

- Murphy, N., Knuppel, A., Papadimitriou, N., Martin, R. M., Tsilifid, K. K., Smith-Byrne, K., . . . Gunter, M. J. (2020, May). Insulin-like growth factor-1, insulin-like growth factor-binding protein-3, and breast cancer risk: Observational and Mendelian randomization analyses with 430,000 women. *Annals of Oncology, 31*(5): 641–649. doi:10.1016/j.annonc.2020.01.066

- Namba, K., Hatano, M., Yaeshima, T., Takase, M., & Suzuki K. (2010). Effects of Bifidobacterium longum BB536 administration on influenza infection, influenza vaccine antibody titer, and cell-mediated immunity in the elderly. *Bioscience, Biotechnology, and Biochemistry, 74*(5): 939–945. doi:10.1271/bbb.90749

- NAMS 2017 Hormone Therapy Position Statement Advisory Panel. (2017). The 2017 hormone therapy position statement of the North American Menopause Society (NAMS). *Menopause, 24*(7): 728–753. doi: 10.1097/GME.0000000000000921

REFERENCES

- National Cancer Institute/National Institutes of Health. (2020). *Home page.* Retrieved from www.nih.gov/.../national-cancer-institute-nci
- National Eye Institute/National Institutes of Health. (2020, April 13). Age-related eye disease studies: AREDS/AREDS2. Retrieved from https://www.nei.nih.gov/research/clinical-trials/age-related-eye-disease-studies-aredsareds2
- National Institutes of Health. (2009, March 19). *Low vitamin D levels associated with colds and flu.* Retrieved from https://www.nih.gov/news-events/nih-research-matters/low-vitamin-d-levels-associated-colds-flu
- National Institutes of Health. (2018, October 10). NIH study finds probiotic Bacillus eliminates Staphylococcus bacteria. (News Release). Bethesda, Maryland: Author. Retrieved from https://www.nih.gov/news-events/news-releases/nih-study-finds-probiotic-bacillus-eliminates-staphylococcus-bacteria.
- National Institutes of Health, Office of Dietary Supplements. (2020a, March 24).

Vitamin D: Fact sheet for health professionals. Retrieved from: https://ods.od.nih.gov/factsheets/VitaminD-HealthProfessional/

- National Institutes of Health, Office of Dietary Supplements. (2020b, April 4). *Zinc: Fact sheet for health professionals*. Retrieved from: https://ods.od.nih.gov/factsheets/Zinc-HealthProfessional/

- National Institute of Mental Health (NIMH). (2019, April). *Suicide*. Retrieved from:

www.nimh.nih.gov/health/statistics/suicide.shtml

- Natural Medicines Comprehensive Database. (n.d.). *Lysine, elderberry, echinacea*. Retrieved from:

http://naturaldatabase.therapeuticresearch.-com/home.aspx?cs=&s=ND

- Natural Medicines Comprehensive Database. (2020). *Home page*. Retrieved from https://naturalmedicines.therapeuticresearch.com/

- Nayeri, A., Wu, S., & Adams, C. (2017).

Acute calcineurin inhibitor nephrotoxicity secondary to turmeric intake: A case report. *Transplantation Proceedings, 49*(1): 198–200.

- Ng, Q. X., Koh, S. S. H., Chan, H. W., & Ho, C. Y. X. (2017, June 1). Clinical Use of Curcumin in Depression: A Meta-Analysis. *Journal of the American Medical Directors Association, 18*(6): 503–508. doi: 10.1016/j.jamda.2016.12.071

- Olivera-Pueya, J., & Pelegrin-Valero, C. (2017, September). Nutritional supplements in anxiety disorder. *Actas Españolas de Psiquiatría, 45*(Supplement): 37–47. Retrieved from https://pubmed.ncbi.nlm.nih.gov/29171642

- Ota, A., & Ulrih, N. P. (2017, July 6). An overview of herbal products and secondary metabolites used for management of type 2 diabetes. *Frontiers of Pharmacology, 8*:4 36. doi:10.3389/fphar.2017.00436

- Pahwa, R., & Jialal, I. (2018, October 27). *Chronic Inflammation.* Retrieved from https://www.ncbi.nlm.nih.gov/books/NBK493173/

- Parikh, S., Saneto, R., Falk, M. J., Anselm, I., Cohen, B. H., Hass, R., & the Mitochondrial Medicine Society. (2009,

October 14). A modern approach to the treatment of mitochondrial disease. *Current Treatment Options in Neurology, 11*(6): 414–430. doi:10.1007/s11940-009-0046-0

- Paul, V., & Ekambaram, P. (2011). Involvement of nitric oxide in learning & memory processes. *Indian Journal of Medical Research*, 133(5): 471–478.

- Pérez-Sánchez, A., Barrajón-Catalán, E., Herranz-López, M., & Micol, V. (2018). Nutraceuticals for skin care: A comprehensive review of human clinical studies. *Nutrients, 10*: 403.

- Perna, S., Alalwan, T. A., Alaali, Z., Alnashaba, T., Gasparri, C., Infantino, V., Hammad, L., . . . Rondanelli, M. (2019, October 22). The role of glutamine in the complex interaction between gut microbiota and health: A narrative review. *International Journal of Molecular Science, 20*(20): 5232. doi:10.3390/ijms20205232

- Piewngam, P., Zheng, Y., Nguyen, T. H., Dickey, S. W., Joo, H. S., Villaruz, A. E., . . . Otto, M. (2018, October 10). Pathogen elimination by probiotic *Bacillus* via signalling interference.

REFERENCES

Nature, 562: 532–537.
doi:10.1038/s41586-018-0616-7

- Pizzorno J. (2014). Mitochondria: Fundamental to life and health. *Integrated Medicine (Encinitas), 13*(2): 8–15.
- Pleschka, S., Stein, M., Schoop, R., & Hudson, J. B. (2009, November 13). Antiviral properties and mode of action of standardized *Echinacea purpurea* extract against highly pathogenic avian influenza virus (H5N1, H7N7) and swine-origin H1N1 (S-OIV). *Virology Journal, 6*: 197. doi:10.1186/1743-422X-6-197
- Poling, J. S., Frye, R. E., Shoffner, J., & Zimmerman, A. W. (2006). Developmental regression and mitochondrial dysfunction in a child with autism. *Journal of Child Neurology*, 21(2): 170–172. doi:10.1177/08830738060210021401
- Poljsak, B. (2016). NAD+ in cancer prevention and treatment: Pros and cons. *Journal of Clinical Experiments in Oncology, 5*:4. doi:10.4172/2324-9110.1000165
- Position of the Academy of Nutrition and Dietetics, Dietitians of Canada, and the American College of Sports Medicine:

Nutrition and athletic performance. (2016, March). *Journal of the Academy of Nutrition and Dietetics, 116*(3): 501–528.

- Prasad, A. S. (2002). Zinc deficiency in patients with sickle cell disease. *American Journal of Clinical Nutrition, 75*:181–182.
- Proudman, J. M., Cleland L. (2010). Fish oil and rheumatoid arthritis: Past, present and future. *Proceedings of the Nutrition Society, 69*: 316–323.
- Pullar, J. M., Carr, A. C., & Vissers, M. C. M. (2017, August 12). The roles of vitamin C in skin health. *Nutrients, 9*(8): 866. doi:10.3390/nu9080866
- Raus, K., Pleschka, S., Klein, P., Schoop, R., & Fish, P. (2015). Effect of an echinacea-based hot drink versus oseltamivir in influenza treatment: a randomized, double-blind, double-dummy, multicenter, noninferiority clinical trial. *Current Therapeutic Research, Clinical and Experimental, 20*(77): 66–72. doi:10.1016/j.curtheres.2015.04.001
- Rechtschaffen, A., & Bergmann, B. M. (2002, February). Sleep deprivation in the rat: An update of the 1989 paper. *Sleep, 25*(1): 18–24.
- Reiter, R. J., Sharma, R., Ma, Q.,

Dominquez-Rodriguez, A., Marik, P. E., & Abreu-Gonzalez, P. (2020, June). Melatonin inhibits Covid-19-induced cytokine storm by reversing aerobic glycolysis in immune cells: A mechanistic analysis. *Medicine in Drug Discovery, 2020*(6): 100044. doi:10.1016/j.medidd.2020.100044

- Richards, J. R., Harms, B. N., Kelly, A., & Turnipseed, S. D. (2018). Methamphetamine use and heart failure: Prevalence, risk factors, and predictors. *American Journal of Emergency Medicine, 36*(8): 1423–1428. doi:10.1016/j.ajem.2018.01.001

- Ridker, P. M. (2019). Anti−inflammatory therapy for atherosclerosis: Interpreting divergent results from the CANTOS and CIRT clinical trials. *Journal of Internal Medicine, 285*: 503–509.

- Rizvi, S., Raza, S. T., Ahmed, F., Ahmad, A., Abbas, S., & Mahdi, F. (2014). The role of vitamin E in human health and some diseases. *Sultan Qaboos University Medical Journal, 14*(2): e157–e165.

- Romagnolo, D. F., Selmin, O. I. (2017). Mediterranean diet and prevention of chronic diseases. *Nutrition Today, 52*(5):

208–222. doi:10.1097/NT.0000000000000228

- Ruggiero, P. (2014). Use of probiotics in the fight against *Helicobacter pylori*. *World Journal of Gastrointestinal Pathophysiology, 5*(4): 384–391. doi: 10.4291/wjgp.v5.i4.384

- Rui, L. (2014). Energy metabolism in the liver. *Comprehensive Physiology, 4*(1): 177–197. doi:10.1002/cphy.c130024

- Sadowska, A. M., Verbraecken, J., Darquennes, K., & DeBacker, W. A. Role of N-acetylcysteine in the management of COPD. (2006). *International Journal of Chronic Obstructive Pulmonary Disease, 1*(4): 425–434. doi:10.2147/copd.2006.1.4.425

- Sears, M. E. (2013, April 18). Chelation: Harnessing and enhancing heavy metal detoxification: A review. *Scientific World Journal, 2013*: Epub. doi:10.1155/2013/219840

- Shaik, M. M., & Gan, S. H. (2015). Vitamin supplementation as possible prophylactic treatment against migraine with aura and menstrual migraine. *Biomedical Research International, 2015*: 469529. doi:10.1155/2015/469529

REFERENCES

- Sharma, A., Gerberg, P. L., & Brown, R. P. (2015). Nonpharmacological treatments for ADHD in youth. *Adolescent Psychiatry (Hilversum)*, 5(2): 84–95. doi:10.2174/2210676605021504301549 37
- Shi, J., Xue, W., Zhao, W. J., & Li, K. X. (2013, February). Pharmacokinetics and dopamine/acetylcholine releasing effects of ginsenoside Re in hippocampus and mPFC of freely moving rats. *Acta Pharmacologica Sinica, 34*: 21420. PMID:23202798. doi:10.1038/ aps.2012.147
- Shils, M., Olson, A., & Shike, M. (1994). *Modern nutrition in health and disease* (8th ed.). Philadelphia, PA: Lea and Febiger.
- Shin, K. K., Yi, Y. S., Kim, J. K., Kim, H., Hossain, M. A., Kim, J. H., & Cho, J. Y. (2020, March 25). Korean red ginseng plays an anti-aging role by modulating expression of aging-related genes and immune cell subsets. *Molecules, 25*(7): 1492. doi:10.3390/molecules25071492
- Shishtar, E., Sievenpiper, J. L., Djedovic, V., Cozma, A. I., Ha, V., Jayalath, V. H., . . . Vuksan, V. (2014, September 29). The effect of ginseng (the genus Panax) on

glycemic control: A systematic review and meta-analysis of randomized controlled clinical trials. *PLOS One*, 9(9):e107391. doi:10.1371/journal.pone.0107391

- Silvestri, M., & Rossi, G. A. (2013, October 3). Melatonin: Its possible role in the management of viral infections: A brief review. *Italian Journal of Pediatrics*, 39: 61. doi:10.1186/1824-7288-39-61

- Sinatra, S. T. (2015). *The Sinatra Solution: Metabolic cardiology* (3rd ed.). North Bergen, NJ: Basic Health Publications.

- Siska, G. (2017, April). *Why I do NOT routinely recommend calcium supplements to maintain strong bones.* Retrieved from:

http://www.pharmacytimes.com/contributor/gunda-siska-pharmd/2017/04/why-i-do-not-routinely-recommend-calcium-supplements-to-maintain-strong-bones

- Siska, G. (2019, November 16). When antivirals are not indicated, natural products can help alleviate flu symptoms. *Pharmacy Times* (online). Retrieved from https://www.pharmacytimes.com/news/when-antivirals-are-not-indicated-natural-products-can-help-alleviate-flu-symptoms

- Souza, D. R., Pieri, B. L. D. S., Comim, V. H., Marques, S. D. O.,Luciano, T. F., Rodrigues, M. S., & Souza, C. T.(2020, January 28). Fish oil reduces subclinical inflammation, insulin resistance, and atherogenic factors in overweight/obese type 2 diabetes mellitus patients: A pre-post pilot study. *Journal of Diabetes Complications*, *34*(5):107553. doi:10.1016/j.jdiacomp.2020.107553
- Stanner, S., Hughes, J., Kelly, C., & Buttriss, J. (2004). Fruits and veggies in diet = better health: A review of the epidemiological evidence for the "antioxidant hypothesis." *Public Health Nutrition, 7*(3), 407–422. doi:10.1079/PHN2003543
- Suliman, N. A., Mat-Taib, C. N., Mohd-Moklas, M. A., Adenan, M. I., Hidayat-Baharuldin, M. T., & Basir, R. (2016). Establishing natural nootropics: Recent Molecular Enhancement Influenced by Natural Nootropics. *Evidence-Based Complementary Alternative Medicine*, *2016*: 4391375. doi:10.1155/2016/4391375
- Surawicz, C. M. (2008). Role of probiotics in antibiotic-associated diarrhea,

Clostridium difficile-associated diarrhea, and recurrent *Clostridium difficile*-associated diarrhea. *Journal of Clinical Gastroenterology, 42*(suppl 2): S64–S70.

- Swan, P. (2005). Goldberger's war: The life and work of a public health crusader. (Review.) *Bulletin of the History of Medicine, 79*(1): 146–147. doi:10.1353/bhm.2005.0046
- Szodoray P, Nakken B., Gaal J., Jonsson, R., Szegedi, A., Zoid, E., Szegedi, G., . . . Bodolay, E. (2008, August 4). The complex role of vitamin D in autoimmune diseases. *Scandinavian Journal of Immunology, 68*(3): 261–269. doi:10.1111/j.1365-3083.2008.02127
- Tangpricha, V. (2016, October 10). Vitamin D deficiency and related disorders. Medscape. Retrieved from http://emedicine.medscape.com/article/128762-overview
- Van Gorkom, G. N. Y., Lookermans, E. L., Van Elssen, C. H. M. J., & Bos, G. M. J. (2019, April 28). The effect of vitamin C (ascorbic acid) in the treatment of patients with cancer: A systematic review. *Nutrients, 11*(5): 977. doi:10.3390/nu11050977

REFERENCES

- Velthuis, A. J., van den Worm, S. H., Sims, A. C., Baric, R. S., Snijder, E. J., & van Hemert, M. J. (2010, November 4). Zn(2+) inhibits coronavirus and arterivirus RNA polymerase activity in vitro, and zinc ionophores block the replication of these viruses in cell culture. *PLOS Pathogens*, *6*(11): e1001176. doi:10.1371/journal.ppat.1001176\

- Vighi, G., Marcucci, F., Sensi, L., Di Cara, G., & Frati, F. (2008). Allergy and the gastrointestinal system. *Clinical and Experimental Immunol*ogy, *153*(Suppl 1): 3–6. doi:10.1111/j.1365-2249.2008.03713.x

- Vitamin C supplementation slightly improves physical activity levels and reduces cold incidence in men with marginal vitamin C status: A randomized controlled trial. (2014). *Nutrients, 6*: 2572–2583.

- Vlachojannis, J. E., Cameron, M., & Chrubasik, S. (2010). A systematic review on the Sambuci fructus effect and efficacy profiles. *Phytotherapy Research, 24(1): 1–8.*

- Wani, A. L., Ara, A., & Usmani, J. A. (2015). Lead toxicity: A review.

Interdisciplinary Toxicology, *8*(2): 55–64. doi:10.1515/intox-2015-0009

- Wu W, Li R, Li X, et al. Quercetin as an Antiviral Agent Inhibits Influenza A Virus (IAV) Entry. *Viruses*. 2015;8(1):6. Published 2015 Dec 25. doi:10.3390/v8010006

- Yeh, T. L., Shih, P. C., Liu, S. J., Lin, C. H., Liu, J. M., & Lei, W. T. (2018, January 25). The influence of prebiotic or probiotic supplementation on antibody titers after influenza vaccination: a systematic review and meta-analysis of randomized controlled trials. *Drug Design, Development, and Therapy*, *12*: 217–230. doi:10.2147/DDDT.S155110

- Yi, J., Horky, L. L., Friedlich, A. L., Shi, Y., Rogers, J. T., & Huang, X. (2009). L-arginine and Alzheimer's disease. *International Journal of Clinical and Experimental Pathology*, *2*(3): 211–238.

- Ziegler, D., Ametov, A., Barinov A., Dyck, P. J., Gurieva, I., Low, P. A., . . . Samigullin, R. (2006). Oral treatment with alpha-lipoic acid improves symptomatic diabetic polyneuropathy: The Sydney 2 Trial. *Diabetes Care, 29*: 2365.

Made in USA - Kendallville, IN
1194302_9798678793201
11.30.2020 1924